ICS 11.020

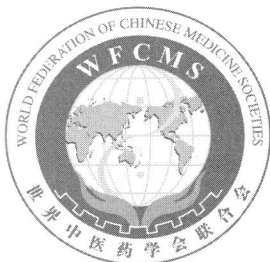

世界中医药学会联合会代谢病专业委员会

Specialty Committee of Metabolic Diseases of WFCMS

Specialty Committee Standard of WFCMS   SCM-C 0014-2019

糖脂代谢病（瘅浊）中西医结合诊疗技术规范

Specification of Diagnosis and Treatment of Glucolipid Metabolic Disorders（Dan-Zhuo）with Integrated Chinese and Western Medicine

世界中联专业（工作）委员会标准   2019-01-11发布实施

图书在版编目（CIP）数据

糖脂代谢病（癉浊）中西医结合诊疗技术规范：汉英对照 / 世界中医药学会联合会代谢病专业委员会编著 . —北京：中国医药科技出版社，2019.6

ISBN 978-7-5214-1216-1

Ⅰ.①糖… Ⅱ.①世… Ⅲ.①糖脂—代谢病—中西医结合—诊疗—技术规范—汉、英 Ⅳ.① R589-65

中国版本图书馆 CIP 数据核字（2019）第 114399 号

美术编辑　陈君杞

版式设计　南博文化

出版　**中国健康传媒集团** | 中国医药科技出版社

地址　北京市海淀区文慧园北路甲 22 号

邮编　100082

电话　发行：010-62227427　邮购：010-62236938

网址　www.cmstp.com

规格　880 × 1230 mm $^1/_{16}$

印张　3 $^3/_4$

字数　94 千字

版次　2019 年 6 月第 1 版

印次　2019 年 6 月第 1 次印刷

印刷　三河市万龙印装有限公司

经销　全国各地新华书店

书号　ISBN 978-7-5214-1216-1

定价　**29.00 元**

获取新书信息、投稿、为图书纠错，请扫码联系我们。

目　次

前　　言

本《规范》的主要起草单位：广东药科大学、首都医科大学附属北京中医医院、中国中医科学院、华中科技大学同济医学院、成都中医药大学附属医院、安徽中医药大学第一附属医院、中山大学附属第一医院、UniMed Center（美国）、Western University（加拿大）。

本《规范》参与起草单位：北京中医药大学、北京中医药大学附属东方医院、北京中医药大学附属东直门医院、北京老年医院、成都中医药大学、复旦大学附属华山医院、甘肃中医药大学、甘肃中医药大学附属医院、广东药科大学附属第一医院、广州华侨医院、广东省中医院、广东省中医药学会、广州医科大学、广州中医药大学第一附属医院、黑龙江省中医药科学院、湖南中医药大学、吉林省中医院、暨南大学中医学院、江西中医药大学附属医院、辽宁中医药大学、南京中医药大学、欧洲经方中医学会（德国）、山东省立医院、山东中医药高等专科学校、陕西中医药大学、陕西中医药大学附属医院、汕头大学医学院附属肿瘤医院、上海市中医药研究院、上海长征医院、上海中医药大学附属岳阳中西医结合医院、深圳市第二人民医院、深圳市中医院、天津市中医药研究院、温州医科大学、云南省中医医院、浙江大学医学院附属第二医院、浙江中医药大学、郑州大学、军事科学院、中国药科大学、中国中医科学院广安门医院、中国中医科学院西苑医院、中山市中医院、重庆医科大学、澳大利亚悉尼健康研究院、澳大利亚中医药学会、欧盟针灸学院（比利时）、美国雅诚健康公司、美国德州奥斯汀中医学院、范德堡大学整合医学中心（美国）、美国圣约翰大学、香港大学、香港大学李嘉诚医学院、香港科技大学、香港中文大学、香港永康制药有限公司。

本《规范》主要起草人：郭姣、张声生、雷燕、陆付耳、谢春光、方朝晖、陶军、刘浩怡（美国）、Subrata Chakrabarti（加拿大）。

本《规范》参与起草人及审阅专家（按姓氏拼音排序）：

中国：别晓东、曹纬国、陈筑红、成福春、邓奕辉、段玉红、范冠杰、范中农、傅南琳、高思华、高月、龚燕冰、何兴祥、胡义扬、焦振山、金玲、金世明、康学东、匡海学、李国标、李惠林、李乐愚、李显筑、李应东、林忠伟、林灼锋、刘建平、刘毅、刘中勇、马毅、朴春丽、朴胜华、荣向路、史大卓、宋宗良、孙慧琳、万海同、王建伟、魏军平、温伟波、吴君、吴宗贵、夏文豪、项磊、徐海波、徐霞、徐艳秋、杨洁红、杨钦河、杨晓晖、杨宇峰、杨震、姚文兵、叶得伟、依秋霞、于心同、余细勇、曾智桓、战丽彬、张广德、张剑勇、张清华、张述耀、张腾、周强、周万兴、朱青、朱章志。

中国香港：冯奕斌、林煌權、倪世明、牛毅、徐爱民、朱翠凤。

美国：陈哲生、何玉信、李子洪、刘浩怡、朱崇兵。

澳大利亚：李育浩、郑建华。

比利时：陶丽玲。

加拿大：Subrata Chakrabarti。

德国：李枫。

本《规范》的起草程序遵守了世界中医药学会联合会发布的SCM 0001-2009《标准制定和发布工作规范》和世界中医药学会联合会秘书处发布的世界中联秘发2011（20号）文件《世界中联各专业委员会专业技术标准制定实施办法》。

引　言

糖脂代谢性疾病包括血糖异常、血脂异常、非酒精性脂肪肝性肝病（NAFLD）、超重、高血压、动脉粥样硬化性心脑血管病等，其发病率居高不下，是世界性难题。

2017年国际糖尿病联盟（International Diabetes Federation, IDF）发布的最新数据显示，全球20~79岁成人糖尿病患病率为8.8%，患病人数约为4.25亿，中国糖尿病患者人数达1.14亿，位居全球第一。此外，血脂异常、NAFLD、超重、高血压等患病率也居高不下，并逐年升高，共同威胁着人类的健康。

近年来，流行病学研究逐渐关注到合病或并病的情况在糖脂代谢性疾病中的危害。2008年，郭姣教授团队首次针对高脂血症患者合病情况展开调查，结果显示高脂血症患者合并糖尿病、高血压等疾病占84.2%。2010~2012年"3B研究"显示，2型糖尿病合并血脂异常、高血压中一种或两种的患者占总人数的72%。与单纯2型糖尿病患者相比，合并血脂异常、高血压的2型糖尿病患者患心血管疾病风险高6倍。而且，研究已证实，糖尿病、血脂异常与非酒精性脂肪性肝病合病会极大增加糖尿病患者微血管并发症和大血管并发症风险。

以上研究说明，糖代谢异常、脂代谢异常、高血压及NAFLD常合病或并病，且相互影响，密切相关，而目前针对糖脂代谢性疾病多采用分科单病诊治的策略，血糖、血脂、血压等综合达标率较低。因此，需要对糖脂代谢性疾病进行综合一体化认识和防控，提高糖脂代谢性疾病综合防控水平。

基于此，广东药科大学郭姣教授率先提出"糖脂代谢病（瘅浊）"的概念，并开展系列研究，得到国内外同行广泛认可，于2015年岭南代谢病国际论坛主导形成糖脂代谢病"广州共识"。鉴于目前尚缺乏糖脂代谢病综合防控的相关标准，为进一步规范糖脂代谢病中西医临床诊断与治疗，为临床实践提供中西医药治疗策略与方法，特制定本《规范》。

糖脂代谢病（瘅浊）中西医结合诊疗技术规范

1 范围

本《规范》规定了糖脂代谢病（瘅浊）的定义、病因病机、诊断标准、辨证论治及综合防控措施的基本要求。

本《规范》适用于各级医疗及科研机构从事糖脂代谢病（瘅浊）中西医结合临床诊疗及科研工作。

2 规范性引用文件

本《规范》无规范性引用文件。

3 术语和定义

下列术语和定义适用于本文件。

3.1

糖脂代谢病

糖脂代谢病是以糖、脂代谢紊乱为特征，由遗传、环境、精神、饮食等多种因素参与致病，以神经内分泌失调、胰岛素抵抗、氧化应激、慢性炎性反应、肠道菌群失调为核心病机，以高血糖、血脂失调、脂肪肝、超重、高血压、动脉粥样硬化等单一或合并出现为主要临床表现，需要从整体上进行综合防控的疾病。

注：糖脂代谢病属于中医"瘅浊"的范畴。

3.2

瘅浊

瘅浊是以情志失调、饮食不节、禀赋不足或年老体衰等为主要原因，以肝失疏泄为上游和枢纽病机，以湿、痰、瘀、热、毒为主要病理产物，以情志抑郁或急躁、形体肥胖或消瘦、头身困重、口苦口黏、胸胁胀闷或疼痛、倦怠乏力、咽干口燥等为主要临床表现的一种病证。

注："瘅"主要指热、湿热、劳病，瘅之为患可损伤全身多个脏腑，包括脾瘅、胃瘅、肾瘅、心瘅、消瘅、肝（胆）瘅等；"浊"指湿、痰、瘀、毒等病理之浊。西医学糖、脂代谢紊乱的病理变化及其产物如高血糖、高脂血症、非酒精性脂肪肝、超重、高血压、动脉粥样斑块等均可归属于"瘅浊"的范畴。

4 发病机制

4.1 西医发病机制

4.1.1 神经－内分泌－免疫紊乱

大脑中的特定神经元可感知代谢底物的变化，并通过与进入脑内的瘦素、胰岛素及其他细胞因子交互作用，综合调节体内的糖脂代谢。

4.1.2 胰岛素抵抗

胰岛素抵抗在糖脂代谢紊乱中起关键作用，肝、脂肪、肌肉、脑等效应器官的胰岛素信号通路受阻，导致对胰岛素敏感性降低，引起全身性糖脂代谢紊乱。

4.1.3 氧化应激

氧化应激是机体内糖脂代谢异常的重要基础。糖毒性与脂毒性均可通过氧化应激损伤胰岛细胞、肌肉、脂肪细胞及其信号通路，引起胰岛素抵抗；同时损伤血管内皮细胞，引起广泛的心脑及外周血管疾病。

4.1.4 慢性炎性反应

慢性炎性反应在糖脂代谢异常的病理中普遍存在。炎性反应因子通过广泛交织的免疫网络，参与调节肝、脂肪、肌肉、胰腺等组织器官的糖、脂代谢功能。因此，通过抗炎治疗糖脂代谢紊乱性疾病也是目前研究关注的重要内容。

4.1.5 肠道菌群失调

肠道菌群对于机体的糖脂代谢具有重要影响。肠道菌群可通过调节炎性反应、调控免疫系统等影响糖脂代谢。因此，肠道菌群紊乱可引发肥胖、高脂血症、糖尿病、动脉粥样硬化等多种代谢性疾病。

4.2 中医病因病机

4.2.1 病因

情志失调；饮食不节，或嗜食肥甘厚腻；禀赋不足，或年老体衰，或劳欲过度。

4.2.2 病位

本病病位主要在肝、脾、肾，后期可涉及心、脑及各脏腑脉络等。

4.2.3 病机

肝失疏泄，五脏六腑皆受其制，水谷津液运化失常，膏脂堆积，日久成瘅（热、湿热、劳病）或酿生湿、痰、瘀、毒诸浊，瘅、浊相互为病，而成"瘅浊"。肝失疏泄为病机的上游和枢纽，湿、痰、瘀、热、毒为主要病理产物。

肝主疏泄，调畅气机，包括调畅情志、助脾胃运化、促进血及津液运行。若长期压力焦虑致情志不舒，则肝气郁滞，气机不畅，肝气横逆乘脾；或饮食不节，嗜食肥甘厚腻，或思虑过多，均可损伤脾胃，导致脾胃虚弱，脾失健运，脾不散精，物不归正化则为痰、为湿；痰湿内结，蕴久化热，痰热自成，积久成毒；肝气郁结，致气滞血瘀，或气滞痰凝，久则痰瘀互结；又气郁化火，火热、痰热耗气伤阴，致气阴两虚；或禀赋不足，或年老体衰，或劳欲过度，或脾病及肾，均可致肾阳不足，不能蒸津化气；又肝气郁滞，血水不利，致水毒泛滥，瘀浊内阻。因此，本病为全身气血津液输布失调，湿、痰、瘀、热、毒诸浊蕴结体内所致。又病变后期，肾元不足，无力温煦、滋养五脏六腑，湿、痰、瘀、热、毒更甚，络脉阻滞与损伤加重，最终多种病理因素共存，多个脏腑同病，虚实夹杂，加重病情，或致缠绵难愈。

5 西医诊断

根据病理进程，糖脂代谢病分为3期，Ⅰ期多无临床症状，仅血液生化指标和/或影像学指标发生轻度改变；Ⅱ期出现相应的临床症状，血液生化指标和/或影像学的改变达到临床诊断标准；Ⅲ期，在Ⅱ期的基础上病情加重，出现并发症。

5.1 糖脂代谢病Ⅰ期

糖脂代谢病Ⅰ期的诊断应符合附录A的规定，且符合以下3条中任何1条或1条以上。

a）糖尿病前期。

b）血脂水平处于边缘升高范围，且有以下2个或2个以上危险因素。

　　1）肥胖，BMI ≥ 28 kg/m²。

　　2）吸烟≥1年，每日≥1支。

　　3）有遗传性家族性高脂血症者。

　　4）有早发性动脉粥样硬化性血管疾病[i]家族史者[ii]。

　　注：i：颈动脉狭窄≥50%、肾动脉狭窄≥50%、下肢动脉硬化闭塞症、冠心病、脑梗塞。ii：指男性一级直系亲属在55岁前或女性一级直系亲属在65岁前患缺血性心血管病。

c）非酒精性单纯性脂肪肝。

5.2 糖脂代谢病Ⅱ期

糖脂代谢病Ⅱ期的诊断应符合附录B的规定，且符合以下4条中任何1条或1条以上。

a）2型糖尿病。

b）血脂异常。

c）非酒精性脂肪性肝炎。

d）有颈动脉或其他动脉粥样硬化斑块，但狭窄<50%。

5.3 糖脂代谢病Ⅲ期

糖脂代谢病Ⅲ期的诊断应符合附录C的规定，且符合以下3条中任何1条或1条以上。

a）糖尿病伴慢性并发症。

b）在糖脂代谢病Ⅱ期基础上并发动脉粥样硬化性血管疾病（颈动脉狭窄≥50%、肾动脉狭窄≥50%、下肢动脉硬化闭塞症、冠心病、脑梗死）。

c）非酒精性脂肪性肝纤维化或肝硬化。

6 中医证候诊断

"瘅浊"主要分为以下七个证型，其中肝郁脾虚证多见于糖脂代谢病Ⅰ期；痰湿阻滞证、湿热内蕴证、气阴两虚证多见于糖脂代谢病Ⅱ期；脾肾阳虚证、痰瘀互结证、阳虚浊毒证多见于糖脂代谢病Ⅲ期。

6.1 肝郁脾虚证

情志抑郁，善太息，劳倦乏力，胸胁胀满或窜痛，纳呆，腹胀，肠鸣矢气，便溏，舌质淡，边有齿痕，苔薄白，脉弦或弦细。

6.2 痰湿阻滞证

头身困重，胸脘痞满，恶心欲吐，善咯痰，口黏腻，纳呆，形体肥胖，舌质淡，舌胖或有齿痕，苔白腻，脉滑或濡。

6.3 湿热内蕴证

脘腹胀闷，面垢油光，口苦，目赤多眵，纳呆厌食，肢体困重，身热不扬，小便短黄，大便黏腻、臭秽不爽，舌红，苔黄腻，脉滑数。

6.4 气阴两虚证

乏力气短，活动后加重，口干，面白少华或颧红，手足心热，失眠多梦，自汗或盗汗，大便秘结，舌质红，少津，苔薄白或少苔，脉细或弱。

6.5 脾肾阳虚证

形寒肢冷，腰膝、腹部冷或冷痛，面色㿠白，面浮肢肿，心悸怔忡，夜尿频多，便质清稀或完谷不化，便次增多或五更泻，舌质淡，舌体胖，边有齿痕，舌苔白滑，脉沉细缓或迟无力。

6.6 痰瘀互结证

胸胁闷痛或刺痛，面色晦暗无华，胸闷脘痞，咯痰，头晕或头痛，语言謇涩，肢体麻木或疼痛，甚或半身不遂，舌紫暗或边有瘀点或瘀斑，苔白或腻，脉弦滑或沉涩。

6.7 阳虚浊毒证

神疲嗜睡，四肢逆冷或周身浮肿，面色黧黑，神识痴呆，咳喘痰多，喘憋气短，恶心或呕吐，腹胀如鼓，腰膝酸软，皮肤瘙痒，肢痿足疽，小便短少，舌质淡，边有齿痕，舌苔浊腻，脉沉迟无力。

7 治疗目标及原则

7.1 治疗目标

针对西医发病机制及中医病因病机进行综合防治，改善糖脂代谢异常，减少或延缓慢性并发症的发生，提高糖脂代谢病有效防控率和临床痊愈水平。

7.2 西医治疗

7.2.1 糖脂代谢病 I 期，以治疗性生活方式改变（Therapeutic Lifestyle Changes,TLC）为主。

a）健康饮食，推荐每日摄入碳水化合物（蔬菜、水果、豆类、全谷类等）占总能量的 50%～65%；摄入脂肪不应超过总能量的 20%～30%，其中饱和脂肪酸摄入量应小于总能量的 7%，反式脂肪酸摄入量应小于总能量的 1%，推荐纤维较高和糖负荷较低的食物，推荐富含单不饱和脂肪酸和多不饱和脂肪酸的地中海式饮食结构。

b）规律运动，每周 5～7 次，每次 30min 中等强度运动。

c）完全戒烟和有效避免吸入二手烟，限制饮酒。

d）保持理想体重，BMI 控制在 20.0～23.9kg/m^2。BMI>35kg/m^2，年龄≥60 岁和有妊娠糖尿病病史的妇女，建议使用二甲双胍预防 2 型糖尿病。

7.2.2 糖脂代谢病 II 期，在治疗性生活方式改变基础上，根据个体动脉硬化性心血管疾病（Arteriosclerotic Cardiovascular Disease, ASCVD）危险程度、血糖情况，进行以调脂、降糖、抗炎保肝为主的治疗。

a）调脂，以降低低密度脂蛋白胆固醇（LDL-C）水平作为防控 ASCVD 危险的首要干预策略。调脂治疗设定的目标值如下：极高危者 LDL-C<1.8mmol/L；高危者 LDL-C<2.6mmol/L；中危和低危者 LDL-C<3.4mmol/L。LDL-C 基线值较高不能达目标值者，LDL-C 至少降低 50%；极高危者 LDL-C 基线在目标值以内者，LDL-C 仍应降低 30% 左右。根据患者情况选择相应的药物，高胆固醇血症、混合性高脂血症者首选以阿托伐他汀为代表的他汀类药物，他汀类药物不能达标者，可联合胆固醇吸收抑制剂，如依折麦布；高甘油三酯血症、甘油三酯（TG）≥5.7mmol/L 者，优先选用贝特类，如非诺贝特；烟酸类或高纯度鱼油制剂亦有降低甘油三酯作用。

b）降糖，血糖的控制参考《American Diabetes Association（2018）》，遵循下面的流程（图1、图2）。

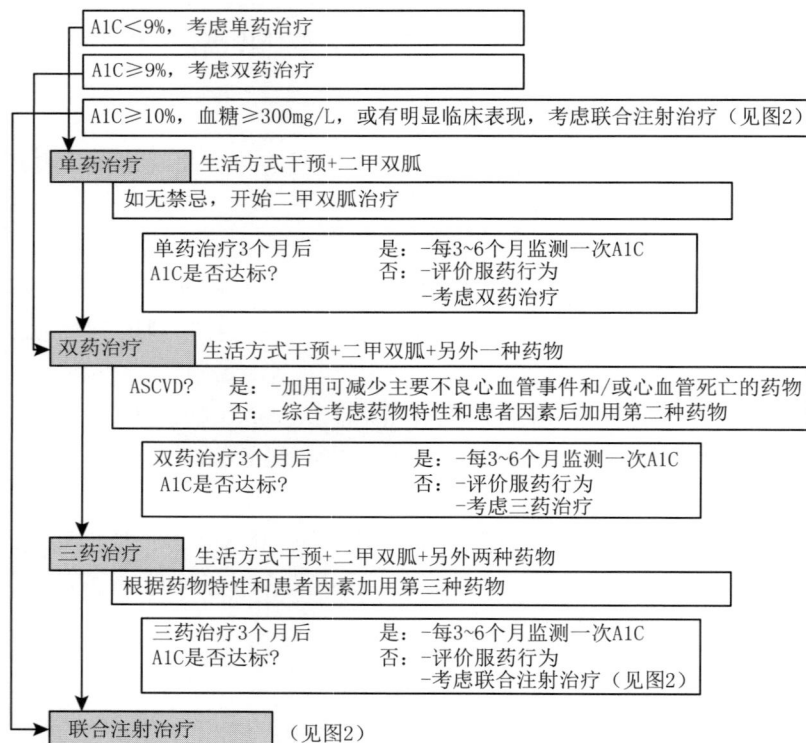

图1 血糖控制的西药治疗原则

开始基础胰岛素
（通常联合二甲双胍+/-其他非胰岛素药物）

开始：每天10U或0.1~0.2U/kg
调整：加量10%~15%或2~4U，每周1次或2次，直至达到空腹血糖目标
针对低血糖：寻找原因并纠正，如果原因不明减量4U或10%~20%

如果A1C控制不佳，考虑联合注射治疗

在食量最大一餐前加用1次速效胰岛素

开始：4U、0.1U/kg或基础剂量的10%，如果A1C＜8%，考虑等量减少基础胰岛素剂量
调整：加量1~2U或10%~15%，每周1次或2次，直至达到自我血糖监测目标
针对低血糖：寻找原因并纠正，如果原因不明，减量2~4U或10%~20%

加用GLP-1受体激动剂

如果不耐受或未达到A1C目标，换用2种胰岛素联合方案

如果未达到目标，考虑换用其他胰岛素方案剂

换用每日2次预混胰岛素（早餐和晚餐前）

开始：将当前基础胰岛素剂量分成2/3a.m.，1/3p.m.或1/2a.m,1/2p.m.
调整：加量1~2U或10%~15%，每周1次或2次，直至达到自我血糖监测目标
针对低血糖：寻找原因并纠正，如果原因不明，减量2~4U或10%~20%

如果A1C控制不佳，开始基础-餐时方案

如果A1C控制不佳，开始每日3次注射方案

餐前加用≥2次速效胰岛素（基础-餐时方案）

开始：每餐4U、0.1U/kg或基础剂量的10%。如果A1C＜8%，考虑等量减少基础胰岛素剂量
调整：加量1~2U或10%~15%，每周1次或2次，直至达到自我血糖监测目标
针对低血糖：寻找原因并纠正，如果原因不明，减量2~4U或10%~20%

如果未达到目标，考虑换用其他胰岛素方案剂

换用每日3次预混胰岛素（早餐、午餐和晚餐前）

开始：在午餐前加用1剂
调整：加量1~2U或10%~15%，每周1次或2次，直至达到自我血糖监测目标
针对低血糖：寻找原因并纠正，如果原因不明，减量2~4U或10%~20%

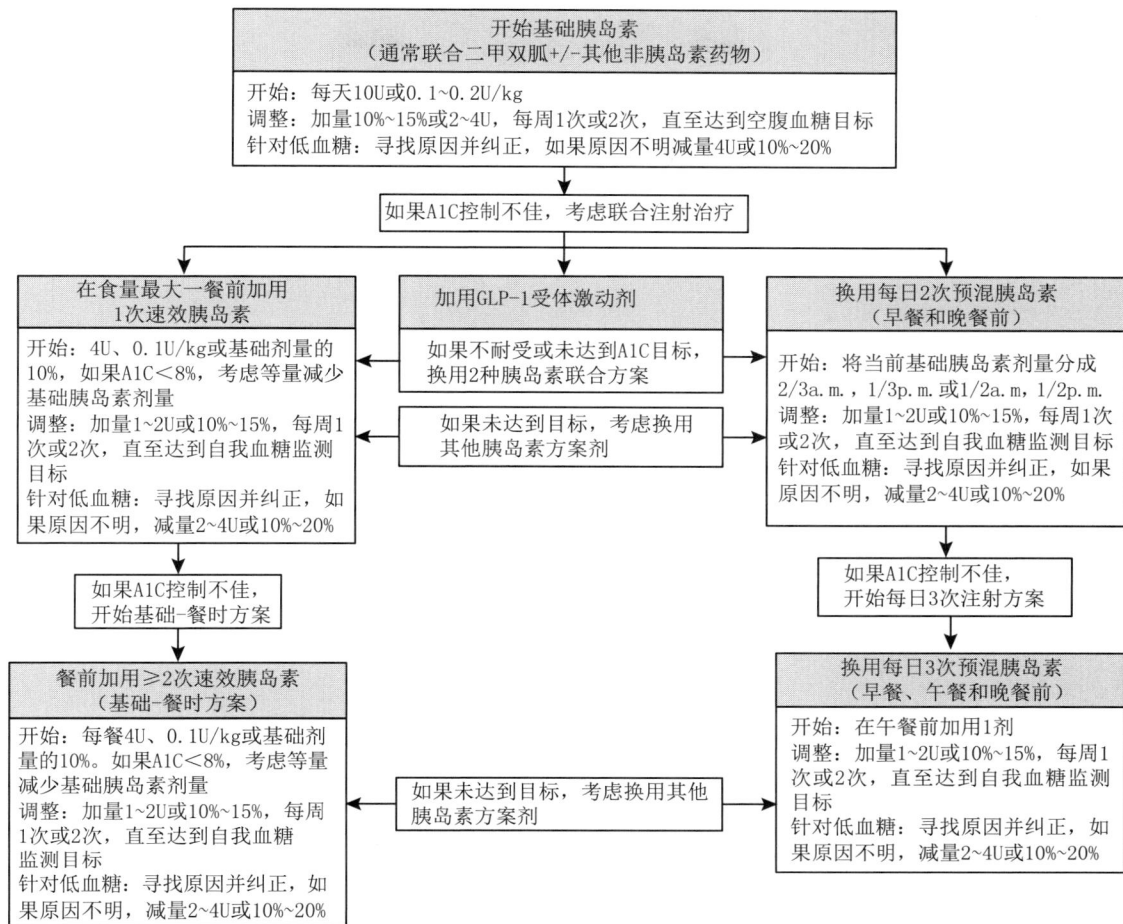

图2 血糖控制的西药联合用药治疗

c）抗炎保肝，有非酒精性脂肪性肝炎的患者，加用抗炎保肝的药物，如双环醇、异甘草酸镁注射液（天晴甘美）等，同时补充益生菌，也可考虑菌群移植治疗。

7.2.3 糖脂代谢病Ⅲ期，针对并发症进行相应治疗。

a）单用他汀类调脂未达标者，首先考虑联合使用胆固醇吸收抑制剂，疗效仍欠佳者可考虑使用新型降脂药物前蛋白转化酶枯草溶菌素9（PSCK9）抑制药如阿里罗单抗等，并在个体化调脂的基础上，严格控制其他高危因素，使用阿司匹林、氯吡格雷等抗血小板药物治疗，防治并发症。

b）相应靶器官动脉严重狭窄甚至闭塞的患者，给予相应的溶栓、球囊扩张或支架植入等治疗。

c）针对糖尿病慢性并发症或者非酒精性脂肪性肝硬化的并发症，在纠正糖脂代谢紊乱的基础上进行相应的对症治疗。

7.3 中医治疗

糖脂代谢病Ⅰ期以肝郁脾虚为主，治以疏肝调畅情志及调理气机升降，兼健脾化浊，增强机体调节气血津液的能力，维持代谢平衡。糖脂代谢病Ⅱ期以虚实夹杂多见，虚证以气阴两虚为主，治以益气养阴；实证以湿、痰、热浊蕴结体内为主，可予调肝舒畅气机，启枢促进运化，兼清热利湿化痰，维持气血津液正常运行，调节诸浊代谢。糖脂代谢病Ⅲ期仍以虚实夹杂为主，虚证以脾肾阳虚为主，治以温补脾肾；实证以痰瘀互结，兼阳虚浊毒、脉络损伤为主要证型，可予祛瘀化痰、化浊解毒。同时严重患者合并有脑、心、肾的衰败，当以各脏腑论治为主。

7.3.1 肝郁脾虚证

［治法］疏肝健脾。

［主方］逍遥散（《太平惠民和剂局方》）加减。

［组成］柴胡、当归、白芍、白术、茯苓、煨生姜、薄荷、炙甘草。

［加减］胁痛重者加丹参、青皮、郁金、佛手；腹胀重者加厚朴、木香；大便稀溏重者加山药、党参、砂仁；心烦易怒加牡丹皮、炒栀子、女贞子。

7.3.2 痰湿阻滞证

［治法］理气化痰祛湿。

［主方］二陈汤合平胃散（《太平惠民和剂局方》）加减。

［组成］二陈汤：姜半夏、陈皮、茯苓、炙甘草；平胃散：苍术、厚朴、橘皮、甘草、生姜、大枣。

［加减］胸胁满闷重者加枳壳、瓜蒌、薤白；喉中痰鸣加胆南星、苏子；头晕明显者加钩藤、天麻、白术；失眠者加夜交藤、远志、胆南星、石菖蒲、茯神。

7.3.3 湿热内蕴证

［治法］清热化湿。

［主方］a）偏中焦选连朴饮（《霍乱论》）加减；b）偏下焦选葛根芩连汤（《伤寒论》）或四妙丸（《成方便读》）加减。

［组成］连朴饮：厚朴、黄连、石菖蒲、制半夏、淡豆豉、焦栀子、芦根；葛根芩连汤：葛根、黄芩、黄连、甘草；四妙丸：川黄柏、薏苡仁、苍术、怀牛膝。

［加减］纳呆厌食者加神曲、连翘、鸡内金；口苦者加柴胡、郁金、茵陈；目赤多眵加龙胆草、夏枯草；小便短黄者加泽泻、大蓟、车前子。

7.3.4 气阴两虚证

［治法］益气养阴。

［主方］参芪地黄汤（《证治宝鉴》）加减。

［组成］人参、黄芪、熟地黄、茯苓、山药、牡丹皮、山茱萸。

［加减］口渴多饮加天花粉、生地、玉竹；自汗盗汗者加浮小麦、煅龙骨、煅牡蛎、五味子；大便秘结者加柏子仁、火麻仁、麦冬；头晕者加钩藤、天麻、半夏；耳鸣重者加石菖蒲、怀牛膝、杜仲；失眠加炒酸枣仁、柏子仁。

7.3.5 脾肾阳虚证

［治法］温补脾肾。

［主方］附子理中丸（《太平惠民和剂局方》）合真武汤（《伤寒论》）加减。

［组成］附子理中丸：炮附子、人参、干姜、炙甘草、白术；真武汤：炮附子、白术、生姜、茯苓、芍药。

［加减］心悸怔忡加肉桂、蛤蚧、五味子；夜尿频多加杜仲、金樱子、芡实；久泄或五更泻加吴茱萸、肉豆蔻、补骨脂；水肿者可加用桂枝、泽泻、猪苓、大腹皮。

7.3.6 痰瘀互结证

［治法］化痰祛瘀。

［主方］瓜蒌薤白半夏汤（《金匮要略》）合血府逐瘀汤《医林改错》）加减。

［组成］血府逐瘀汤：桃仁、红花、当归、生地黄、牛膝、川芎、桔梗、赤芍、枳壳、甘草、柴胡；瓜蒌薤白半夏汤：瓜蒌、薤白、半夏、白酒。

［加减］肢体麻木、疼痛重者加田三七、鸡血藤、桂枝、地龙；喉中痰鸣加石菖蒲、化橘红、浙贝母；脘腹痞闷者加枳实、厚朴；头痛重者加地龙、全蝎、细辛。

7.3.7 阳虚浊毒证

［治法］温阳化浊。

［主方］温脾汤（《备急千金要方》）加减。

［组成］附子、大黄、当归、干姜、人参、甘草。

［加减］喘憋气促重者加炙麻黄、杏仁、丹参、田三七；呕恶重者加吴茱萸、黄连、生姜；皮肤瘙痒者加蛇蜕、当归、地肤子、白鲜皮外洗；小便短少加桂枝、泽泻、茯苓。

此期患者病情危重，应充分发挥中西医各自治疗优势，必要时针对相应器官的功能障碍，采用保肝、强心、护肾等西医治疗手段。

8 综合防控措施

除上述中、西医治疗外，本病还可以加用针灸、热敷、推拿等疗法，同时注重饮食控制、运动、减重等健康管理方式，辅以心理调护等，综合控制糖脂代谢病的发生与发展。

附录 A

（规范性附录）

糖脂代谢病Ⅰ期诊断方法

A.1 糖尿病前期（IGT/IFG）诊断标准

参考《WHO 糖尿病诊断标准，1999》。

在糖尿病出现之前，有一段胰岛素抵抗和胰岛 β 细胞损伤的时期，称为糖尿病前期，此时血糖水平高于正常，但尚未达到目前的糖尿病诊标准，也称为糖调节受损（Impaired Glucose Regulation, IGR）。根据空腹和负荷后血糖值，IGR 可分为两种高血糖状态：空腹血糖受损（Impaired Fasting Glucose, IFG）和糖耐量异常（Impaired Glucose Tolerance, IGT）。

表 A.1 WHO 1999 糖尿病前期分类

	空腹血糖（mmol/L）	餐后 2h 血糖（mmol/L）
空腹血糖受损（IFG）	>6.1 且 <7.0	<7.8
糖耐量异常（IGT）	<6.1	>7.8 且 <11.1
IFG+IGT	>6.1 且 <7.0	>7.8 且 <11.1

A.2 血脂边缘升高范围

参考中国成人血脂异常防治指南修订联合委员会修订的《中国成人血脂异常防治指南（2016年修订版）》。

表 A.2 血脂合适水平和异常分层标准［mmol/L（mg/dl）］

分层	TC	LDL-C	HDL-C	非-HDL-C	TG
理想水平		<2.6（100）		<3.4（130）	
合适水平	<5.2（200）	<3.4（130）		<4.1（160）	<1.7（150）
边缘升高	≥5.2（200）且 <6.2（240）	≥3.4（130）且 <4.1（160）		≥4.1（160）且 <4.9（190）	≥1.7（150）且 <2.3（200）
升高	≥6.2（240）	≥4.1（160）		≥4.9（190）	≥2.3（200）
降低			<1.0（40）		

注：TC：总胆固醇；LDL-C：低密度脂蛋白胆固醇；HDL-C：高密度脂蛋白胆固醇；非-HDL-C：非高密度脂蛋白胆固醇；TG：甘油三酯。

A.3 非酒精性单纯性脂肪肝诊断标准

a）无饮酒史或饮酒折合乙醇量小于 140 g/周（女性 <70 g/周）。

b）除外病毒性肝炎、药物性肝病、全胃肠外营养、肝豆状核变性、自身免疫性肝病等可导致脂肪肝的特定疾病。

c）肝活检组织学改变符合脂肪性肝病的病理学诊断标准，且活动度积分<3分。

表A.3　肝穿刺活检评估 NAFLD 活动度的评估标准（NAFLD activity score，NAS）

病理改变	评分			
	0分	1分	2分	3分
肝细胞脂肪变	<5%	5%~33%	34%~66%	>66%
小叶内慢性炎性反应（20倍镜计数坏死灶）	无	<2个	2~4个	>4个
肝细胞气球样变	无	少见	多见	

鉴于肝组织学诊断难以获得，非酒精性单纯性脂肪肝定义为：肝脏影像学表现符合弥漫性脂肪肝的诊断标准且无其他原因可供解释（Fibro-Touch：240db/m ≤ 脂肪衰减值<265db/m 轻度，265db/m ≤ 脂肪衰减值<295db/m 中度，295db/m ≤ 脂肪衰减值，重度脂肪肝），且外周血肝生化指标正常。

此外，多数患者HOMA指数超过0.5，存在胰岛素抵抗（IR）。可有肠道菌群失调，甲烷氢呼气检查 H^2、CH^4 呼气高峰值提前出现或峰值升高。

附录 B
（规范性附录）
糖脂代谢病Ⅱ期诊断方法

B.1　2 型糖尿病的诊断标准

参考《WHO糖尿病诊断标准，1999》。

表B.1　WHO 2型糖尿病诊断标准，1999

诊断标准	静脉血浆葡萄糖水平（mmol/L）
典型糖尿病症状（多饮、多尿、多食、体重下降）加上随机血糖检测	≥11.1
或加上	
FPG检测	≥7.0
或加上	
葡萄糖负荷后2h血糖检测	≥11.1
无糖尿病症状者，需改日重复检查	

注：a. 空腹状态指至少8h未进食热量。

b. 随机血糖指不考虑上次用餐时间，一天中任意时间的血糖，不能用来诊断空腹血糖受损或糖耐量异常。

c. 葡萄糖负荷后2h血糖检测：口服葡萄糖（75g 脱水葡萄糖）耐量试验（OGTT）中2h 的血浆葡萄糖（2h PG）水平。

d. 2010年ADA指南将HbA1c≥6.5%作为糖尿病诊断标准之一，2011年WHO也建议在条件具备的国家和地区采用这一切点诊断糖尿病。但鉴于HbA1c检测在我国尚不普遍，检测方法的标准化程度不够，缺乏我国人群的HbA1c的大样本研究，所以本标准仍不推荐采用HbA1c作为诊断2型糖尿病（T2DM），但可作为治疗情况的监测指标。

B.2　血脂异常诊断标准

参考中国成人血脂异常防治指南修订联合委员会修订的《中国成人血脂异常防治指南（2016年修订版）》。

表B.2　血脂异常临床分类

	TC	TG	HDL-C	相当于WHO表型
高胆固醇血症	增高			Ⅱa
高TG血症		增高		Ⅳ、Ⅰ
混合型高脂血症	增高	增高		Ⅱb、Ⅲ、Ⅳ、Ⅴ
低HDL-C血症			降低	

注：TC：总胆固醇；TG：甘油三酯；HDL-C：高密度脂蛋白胆固醇。

由于血脂异常的主要危害是增加动脉粥样硬化性心血管疾病（ASCVD）的发病危险，根据《中国成人血脂异常防治指南（2016年修订版）》，ASCVD发病总体危险的评估方法和危险分层的标准如下。

B.2.1　符合下列任意条件者，可直接列为高危ASCVD人群。

　　a）LDL-C≥4.9mmol/L，或TC≥7.2mmol/L。

　　b）年龄≥40岁的糖尿病患者，1.8mmol/L≤LDL-C<4.9mmol/L，或3.1mmol/L≤TC<7.2mmol/L。

B.2.2　不具有以上情况的个体，在考虑是否需要调脂治疗同时，应按照下表B.3进行未来10年间ASCVD总体发病危险的评估，不同组合的ASCVD 10年发病平均危险按<5%，5%~9%，≥10%分别定义为低危、中危和高危。

表B.3　ASCVD发病危险的评估

危险因素 * 个数		血清胆固醇水平分层（mmol/L）		
		3.1≤TC<4.1 或 1.8≤LDL-C<2.6	4.1≤TC<5.2 或 2.6≤LDL-C<3.4	5.2≤TC<7.2 或 3.4≤LDL-C<4.9
无高血压	0~1	低危	低危	低危
	2	低危	低危	中危
	3	低危	中危	中危
有高血压	0	低危	低危	低危
	1	低危	中危	中危
	2	中危	高危	高危
	3	高危	高危	高危

　　注：危险因素包括吸烟、低HDL-C、男性≥45岁或女性≥55岁。

B.2.3　对于ASCVD 10年发病危险为中危的人群进行ASCVD余生危险的评估，以识别出中青年ASCVD余生危险为高危的个体，对包括血脂在内的危险因素进行早期干预。对于ASCVD 10年发病危险为中危的人群，如果具有以下任意2项及以上危险因素，其ASCVD余生危险为高危。这些危险因素包括以下几点。

　　a）收缩压≥160mmHg（1mmHg=0.133kPa）或舒张压≥100mmHg。

　　b）非HDL-C≥5.2mmol/L（200mg/dl）。

　　c）HDL-C<1.0mmol/L（40mg/dl）。

　　d）体质量指数（BMI）≥28kg/m^2。

　　e）吸烟。

B.3　非酒精性脂肪性肝炎的诊断标准

在诊断非酒精性单纯脂肪性肝病的基础上，且肝生化指标异常或者肝穿刺活检评估NAS>4分，可伴有糖尿病前期或血脂边缘升高。多数患者HOMA指数超过0.5，存在IR。多数有肠道菌群失调，甲烷氢呼气检查H^2、CH^4呼气高峰值提前出现或峰值升高。

附录 C
（规范性附录）
糖脂代谢病Ⅲ期诊断方法

C.1 糖尿病慢性并发症的诊断标准

C.1.1 糖尿病肾病

参考中华医学会糖尿病学分会修订的《中国2型糖尿病防治指南（2013版）》。

a）Ⅰ期：肾小球高滤过，肾脏体积增大。

b）Ⅱ期：间断微量白蛋白尿，患者休息时晨尿或随机尿白蛋白与肌酐比值（ACR）正常（男 <2.5mg/mmol，女 <3.5mg/mmol），病理检查可发现肾小球基底膜（GBM）轻度增厚及系膜基质轻度增宽。

c）Ⅲ期：早期糖尿病肾病期，以持续性微量白蛋白尿为标志，ACR为 2.5～30.0mg/mmol（男），3.5～30.0mg/mmol（女），病理检查GBM增厚及系膜基质增宽明显，小动脉壁出现玻璃样变。

d）Ⅳ期：临床糖尿病肾病期，显性蛋白尿，ACR>30.0mg/mmol，部分可表现为肾病综合征，病理检查肾小球病变更重，部分肾小球硬化，灶状肾小管萎缩及间质纤维化。

e）Ⅴ期：肾衰竭期。

C.1.2 糖尿病视网膜病变

参考美国眼科学会编写的《糖尿病视网膜病变（2017更新版）》。

糖尿病视网膜病变是糖尿病高度特异性的微血管并发症，在20～74岁成人新发失明病例中，糖尿病视网膜病变是最常见的病因。糖尿病视网膜病变依据散瞳后检眼底镜下可观察的指标来分级，国际临床分级标准如表C.1。

表C.1 糖尿病视网膜病变国际临床分级

病变严重水平	散瞳后眼底镜下表现
无明显糖尿病视网膜病变	无异常
轻度NPDR	仅有微血管瘤
中度NPDR	比微血管瘤更严重，但程度轻于重度NPDR
重度NPDR	
AAO定义	下列各项中的任何一项，并无增殖性视网膜病变表现： ·在四个象限中每个象限均有严重的视网膜内出血及微血管瘤 ·在两个或更多象限中有明确的静脉串珠样改变 ·在一个或多个象限中有中度IRMA
国际定义	下列各项中的任何一项，并无增殖性视网膜病变表现： ·在四个象限中每个象限均有20处以上的视网膜内出血 ·在两个或更多象限中有明确的静脉串珠样改变 ·在一个或多个象限中有显著IRMA
PDR	具有下列两项中的一项或两项： ·新生血管形成 ·玻璃体/视网膜积血

注：NPDR：非增殖期视网膜病变；AAO：美国眼科学会；PDR：增殖期视网膜病变。

C.1.3 糖尿病并发心血管病变

冠心病风险评估：对所有糖代谢异常的患者应注意询问有无冠心病的症状，有症状者及时进行相关检查及治疗；无症状心肌缺血的筛查手段包括心电图运动负荷试验、动态心肌显像或负荷超声心动图等，应根据患者的具体情况选用，单独动态心电图不能诊断无症状心肌缺血。上述检查提示无症状心肌缺血者，可酌情进行冠状动脉CT血管造影（CTA）并计算钙化积分，有利于预测预后和进一步选择治疗手段。

C.1.4 糖尿病并发脑血管病变

卒中风险评估：糖尿病是卒中的独立危险因素，尤其是缺血性脑血管病。与冠心病的评估筛查原则一样，重点为神经系统症状、体征及恰当的辅助检查来综合评估，包括同型半胱氨酸、颈动脉及经颅多普勒超声、头颅CT、磁共振及血管成像，部分患者需要进行心血管相关检查，以筛查高危心源性栓塞患者。糖尿病患者是颈动脉病变的高危人群，而颈动脉病变是卒中发生的独立危险因素，应重视颈动脉听诊作为颈动脉狭窄的初筛手段。借助颅内外血管超声、头部CT或磁共振及血管成像手段早期发现糖尿病患者无症状性颈动脉病变或无症状性脑梗死。

C.1.5 糖尿病合并外周血管病变

参考中华医学会糖尿病学分会修订的《中国2型糖尿病防治指南（2017年版）》。

糖尿病外周血管病变通常是指下肢动脉性病变（Peripheral Artery Disease, PAD），由于下肢血管的动脉粥样硬化而导致动脉的狭窄、闭塞，严重者可发生下肢远端组织缺血坏死。PAD作为全身动脉硬化的一个标志，常与其他大血管并发症并存。诊断应符合如下标准。

a）如果患者静息踝肱指数（Ankle Brachial Index, ABI）≤0.90，无论患者有无下肢不适的症状。

b）运动时出现下肢不适且静息ABI≥0.90的患者，如踏车平板试验后ABI下降15%~20%；如果患者静息ABI<0.40或踝动脉压<50mmHg或趾动脉压<30mmHg，应该诊断严重肢体缺血。

C.1.6 糖尿病远端对称性多发性神经病变

参考中华医学会糖尿病学分会修订的《中国2型糖尿病防治指南（2017年版）》。

C.1.6.1 糖尿病远端对称性多发性神经病变的诊断标准

a）明确的糖尿病病史。

b）诊断糖尿病时或之后出现的神经病变。

c）临床症状和体征与糖尿病远端对称性多发性神经病变的表现相符。

d）有临床症状（疼痛、麻木、感觉异常等）者，5项检查（踝反射、针刺痛觉、震动觉、压力觉、温度觉）中任1项异常。

e）无临床症状者，5项检查中任2项异常，临床诊断为糖尿病远端对称性多发性神经病变。

C.1.6.2 糖尿病远端对称性多发性神经病变的排除诊断

a）排除其他病因引起的神经病变，如颈腰椎病变（神经根压迫、椎管狭窄、颈腰椎退行性变）、脑梗死、吉兰-巴雷综合征。

b）排除严重动静脉血管性病变，如静脉栓塞、淋巴管炎。

c）尚需鉴别药物尤其是化疗药物引起的神经毒性作用以及肾功能不全引起的代谢毒物对神经的损伤。

d）需要进行鉴别诊断的患者，可做神经肌电图检查。

C.1.6.3 糖尿病远端对称性多发性神经病变的临床诊断分层

C.1.6.3.1 确诊：有糖尿病远端对称性多发性神经病变的症状或体征，同时存在神经传导功能异常。

C.1.6.3.2 临床诊断：有糖尿病远端对称性多发性神经病变的症状及1项体征为阳性，或无症状但有2项以上（含2项）体征为阳性。

C.1.6.3.3 疑似：有糖尿病远端对称性多发性神经病变的症状但无体征，或无症状但有1项体征阳性。

C.1.6.3.4 亚临床：无症状和体征，仅存在神经传导功能异常。

C.1.6.4 糖尿病性自主神经病变

C.1.6.4.1 心血管自主神经病变：表现为直立性低血压、晕厥、冠状动脉舒缩功能异常、无痛性心肌梗死、心脏骤停或猝死。目前尚无统一诊断标准，检查项目包括心率变异性、Valsalva试验、握拳试验（持续握拳3min后测血压）、体位性血压变化测定、24h动态血压监测、频谱分析等。

C.1.6.4.2 消化系统自主神经病变：表现为吞咽困难、呃逆、上腹饱胀、胃部不适、便秘、腹泻及排便障碍等。检查项目可选用胃电图、食管测压、胃排空的闪烁图扫描（测定固体和液体食物排空的时间）及直肠局部末梢神经病变的电生理检查，有助于诊断。

C.1.6.4.3 泌尿生殖系统自主神经病变：临床出现排尿障碍、尿潴留、尿失禁、尿路感染、性欲减退、勃起功能障碍、月经紊乱等。超声检查可判定膀胱容量、残余尿量，神经传导速度检查可以确定糖尿病尿道-神经功能。

C.1.6.4.4 其他自主神经病变：如体温调节和出汗异常，表现为出汗减少或不出汗，从而导致手足干燥开裂，容易继发感染。另外，由于毛细血管缺乏自身张力，致静脉扩张，易在局部形成"微血管瘤"而继发感染。对低血糖反应不能正常感知等。

C.1.7 糖尿病下肢血管病变的诊断

参考中华医学会糖尿病学分会修订的《中国2型糖尿病防治指南（2017年版）》，诊断标准如下。

a）符合糖尿病诊断。

b）具有下肢缺血的临床表现。

c）辅助检查提示下肢血管病变。静息时ABI<0.9，或静息时ABI>0.9，但运动时出现下肢不适症状，行踏车平板试验后ABI降低15%~20%或影像学提示血管存在狭窄。

C.1.8 糖尿病周围神经病变的诊断

参考中华医学会糖尿病学分会修订的《中国2型糖尿病防治指南（2017年版）》，诊断标准如下。

a）明确的糖尿病病史。

b）在诊断糖尿病时或之后出现的神经病变。

c）临床症状和体征与糖尿病周围神经病变的表现相符。

d）以下5项检查中如果有2项或2项以上异常则诊断为糖尿病周围神经病变。

　　1）温度觉异常。

　　2）尼龙丝检查提示足部感觉减退或消失。

　　3）震动觉异常。

　　4）踝反射消失。

　　5）神经传导速度有2项或2项以上减慢。

C.2 急性冠状动脉综合征（ACS）

急性冠状动脉综合征（ACS）是以冠状动脉粥样硬化斑块破裂或侵袭，继发完全或不完全闭塞性血栓形成为病理基础的一组临床综合征，包括急性ST段抬高性心肌梗死（STEMI）、急性非ST段抬高性心肌梗死（NSTEMI）和不稳定型心绞痛（UA），其诊断标准如下。

表C.2　ACS的分类及诊断标准

ACS分类	诊断标准
STEMI	cTn>99thULN 或 CK-MB>99thULN，心电图表现为ST段弓背向上抬高，伴有下列情况之一或以上者：持续性缺血性胸痛（时间超过30min，舌下含服硝酸甘油不能缓解）；超声心动图显示节段性室壁运动异常；冠状动脉造影异常
NSTEMI	cTn>99thULN 或 CK-MB>99thULN，并同时伴有下列情况之一或以上者：持续性缺血性胸痛（时间超过30min，舌下含服硝酸甘油不能缓解）；心电图表现为新发的ST段压低或T波低平、倒置；超声心动图显示节段性室壁运动异常；冠状动脉造影异常
UA	cTn阴性，缺血性胸痛（新出现，或发作较前频繁，或持续时间延长，或程度加重，或在休息时及夜间发作），心电图表现为一过性ST段压低或T波低平、倒置，少见ST段抬高（变异性心绞痛）

注：cTn：肌钙蛋白；CK-MB：肌酸磷化酶-同功酶MB；ULN：正常参考值上限；心电图表现为ST段弓背向上抬高：至少两个相邻导联J点后新出现ST段弓背向上抬高（V2-V3导联 ≥ 0.25mV（<40岁男性）、 ≥ 0.20mV（ ≥ 40岁男性）或 ≥ 0.15mV（女性），其他相邻胸导联或肢体导联 ≥ 0.1mV伴或不伴病理性Q波、R波减低。

C.3　稳定型心绞痛

a）典型劳累性心绞痛病史半年以上。

b）发病时心电图出现ST-T改变。

c）冠状动脉造影显示至少一支血管存在 ≥ 50%的固定性狭窄。

C.4　急性缺血性脑卒中（急性脑梗死）

a）急性起病。

b）局灶神经功能缺损（一侧面部或肢体无力或麻木、言语障碍等），少数为全面神经功能缺损。

c）症状或体征持续时间不限（当影像学显示有责任缺血性病灶时），或持续24小时以上（当缺乏影像学责任病灶时）。

d）排除非血管性病因。

e）脑CT或MRI排除脑出血。

C.5　短暂性脑缺血发作（TIA）

脑、脊髓或视网膜局灶性缺血所致的、未发生急性脑梗死的短暂性神经功能障碍。

C.6　周围动脉疾病（PAD）

指除冠状动脉和颅内动脉以外的动脉疾病，包括动脉狭窄、动脉闭塞和动脉瘤疾病。这些病变主要与动脉硬化相关，慢性炎性反应性、遗传性发育不良和创伤性周围动脉疾病仅占所有PAD病例的5%~10%。

C.7　非酒精性脂肪性肝硬化诊断标准

a）有非酒精性单纯脂肪性肝病的病史。

b）B超和/或CT检查提示肝硬化或者Fibro-Touch检查肝脏硬度 ≥ 11.9kPa，或者肝活检显微镜下可见假小叶形成、纤维组织增生。

c）处于该阶段的患者可有小肠细菌过度生长，且多伴有肠道屏障功能受损。

C.8 下肢动脉硬化闭塞症的诊断标准

符合下述诊断标准前4条可以做出下肢ASO的临床诊断。

a）年龄>40岁。

b）有吸烟、糖尿病、高血压、高脂血症等高危因素。

c）有下肢动脉硬化闭塞症的临床表现。

d）缺血肢体远端动脉搏动减弱或消失。

e）ABI ≤ 0.9。

f）彩色多普勒超声、CTA、MRA和DSA等影像学检查显示相应动脉的狭窄或闭塞等病变。

参 考 文 献

［1］ 国家技术监督局.中医临床诊疗术语 疾病部分［S］.北京：中国标准出版社，GB/T16751.1—1997.

［2］ 国家技术监督局.中医临床诊疗术语 证候部分［S］.北京：中国标准出版社，GB/T16751.2—1997.

［3］ 国家技术监督局.中医临床诊疗术语 治法部分［S］.北京：中国标准出版社，GB/T16751.3—1997.

［4］ 中华中医药学会.中医内科常见病诊疗指南 中医病证部分［S］.北京：中国中医药出版社，ZYYXH/T41—2008.

［5］ 中华中医药学会.中医内科常见病诊疗指南 西医疾病部分［S］.北京：中国中医药出版社，ZYYXH/T50-135—2008.

［6］ 中华中医药学会.糖尿病中医防治指南 糖尿病及其并发症部分［S］.北京：中国中医药出版社，ZYYXH/T3.1-15—2007.

［7］ 郭姣，肖雪，荣向路，等.糖脂代谢病与精准医学［J］.世界科学技术-中医药现代化，2017,19（1）:50-54.

［8］ Guo J.Research progress on prevention and treatment of glucolipid metabolic disease with integrated traditional Chinese and Western medicine［J］.Chin J Integr Med,2017,23（6）:403-409.

［9］ International Diabetes Federation.IDF Diabetes Atlas.8th ed.［EB/OL］.https://www.idf.org/e-library/welcome.html,2017/2018-09-10.

［10］ Wang L,Gao P,Zhang M,et al.Prevalence and Ethnic Pattern of Diabetes and Prediabetes in China in 2013［J］.JAMA,2017,317（24）:2515-2523.

［11］ 国家卫生和计划生育委员会疾病预防控制局.中国居民营养与慢性病状况报告（2015年）［R］.北京:人民卫生出版社，2015.

［12］ Moran A,Gu D,Zhao D,et al.Future Cardiovascular Disease in China:Markov Model and Risk Factor Scenario Projections From the Coronary Heart Disease Policy Model-China［J］.Circulation:Cardiovascular Quality and Outcomes,2010,3（3）:243-252.

［13］ Younossi ZM,Koenig AB,Abdelatif D,et al.Global epidemiology of nonalcoholic fatty liver disease-Meta-analytic assessment of prevalence,incidence,and outcomes［J］.Hepatology, 2016, 64（1）:73-84.

［14］ 项磊，朴胜华，荣向路，等.湿热证病证分布规律探析［J］.世界中医药，2018，13（10）:2621-2624.

［15］ 中华医学会糖尿病学分会.中国2型糖尿病防治指南［S］.北京:北京大学医学出版社，2014.

［16］ 方朝晖，仝小林，段俊国，等.糖尿病前期中医药循证临床实践指南［J］.中医杂志,2017,58（3）:266-270.

［17］ 中华中医药学会糖尿病分会.糖尿病合并代谢综合征中医诊疗标准［J］.世界中西医结合杂志，2011，6（2）:177-179.

［18］ 中国成人血脂异常防治指南修订联合委员会.中国成人血脂异常防治指南（2016年修订版）［J］.中国循环杂志，2016，31（10）:937-950.

［19］ 中国中西医结合学会心血管病专业委员会动脉粥样硬化与血脂异常专业组.血脂异常中西医结合诊疗专家共识［J］.中国全科医学，2017，20（3）:262-269.

［20］ 中华医学会肝病学分会脂肪肝和酒精性肝病学组，中国医师协会脂肪性肝病专家委员会.非酒精性脂肪性肝病防治指南（2018年更新版）［J］.实用肝脏病杂志，2018，21（2）:177-186.

［21］ 中华中医药学会脾胃病分会.非酒精性脂肪性肝病中医诊疗专家共识意见（2017）［J］.中医杂志，2017，58（19）:1706-1710.

［22］ Chalasani N,Younossi Z,Lavine JE,et al.The diagnosis and management of non-alcoholic fatty liver disease:practice Guideline by the American Association for the Study of Liver Diseases,American College of

Gastroenterology,and the American Gastroenterological Association[J].Hepatology,2012,55(6):2005-2023.

［23］ Wong VW,Chan WK,Chitturi S,et al.Asia-Pacific Working Party on Non-alcoholic Fatty Liver Disease guidelines 2017-Part 1:Definition,risk factors and assessment［J］.J Gastroenterol Hepatol,2018,33（1）:70-85.

［24］ Robinson JG,Stone NJ.The 2013 ACC/AHA guideline on the treatment of blood cholesterol to reduce atherosclerotic cardiovascular disease risk: a new paradigm supported by more evidence［J］.Eur Heart J,2015,36（31）:2110-2118.

［25］ 史大卓.冠心病血瘀证诊断标准［J］.中国中西医结合杂志，2016，36（10）:1162-1162.

［26］ 中国医师协会急诊医师分会，中华医学会心血管病学分会，中华医学会检验医学分会.急性冠脉综合征急诊快速诊疗指南［J］.中华急诊医学杂志，2016，25（4）:397-404.

［27］ 中华医学会神经病学分会脑血管病学组急性缺血性脑卒中诊治指南撰写组.中国急性缺血性脑卒中诊治指南2010［J］.中华神经科杂志，2010，43（2）:146-153.

［28］ 北京市脑卒中诊疗质量控制与改进中心.脑动脉粥样硬化筛查与诊断规范（2014版）［J］.中华医学杂志，2014，94（47）:3705-3711.

［29］ 安冬青，吴宗贵.动脉粥样硬化中西医结合诊疗专家共识［J］.中国全科医学，2017，20（5）:507-511.

［30］ 中华医学会外科学分会血管外科学组.颈动脉狭窄诊治指南［J］.中国血管外科杂志（电子版），2017，9（3）:169-175.

［31］ 动脉粥样硬化性肾动脉狭窄诊治中国专家建议（2010）写作组，中华医学会老年医学分会，《中华老年医学杂志》编辑委员会.动脉粥样硬化性肾动脉狭窄诊治中国专家建议（2010）［J］.中华老年医学杂志，2010，29（4）:265-270.

［32］ 中华医学会外科学分会血管外科学组.下肢动脉硬化闭塞症诊治指南（上）［J］.中国血管外科杂志（电子版），2015，7（3）:145-151.

［33］ 郑筱萸.中药新药临床研究指导原则（试行)［M］.北京:中国医药科技出版社，2002.

［34］ Zhai HL,Wang NJ,Han B,et al.Low vitamin D levels and non-alcoholic fatty liver disease,evidence for their independent association in men in East China: a cross-sectional study［Survey on Prevalence in East China for Metabolic Diseases and Risk Factors（SPECT-China）］［J］.Br J Nutr,2016,115（8）:1352-1359.

［35］ Bovet P,Chiolero A,Gedeon J.Health Effects of Overweight and Obesity in 195 Countries［J］.N Engl J Med,2017,377（15）:1495-1496.

［36］ World Health Organization,A global brief on Hypertension［EB/OL］. https://www.who.int/ cardiovascular_ diseases/publications/global_brief_hypertension/zh,2013/2018-10-14.

［37］ Wang Z,Chen Z,Zhang L,et al.Status of Hypertension in China: Results from the China Hypertension Survey,2012-2015［J］.Circulation, 2018,137（22）:2344-2356.

［38］ Yu X,Tian X,Wang S.Age-specific relevance of usual blood pressure to vascular mortality: a meta-analysis of individual data for one million adults in 61 propective studies［J］.Journal of the Lepidopterists Society,2002,52（26）:141-147.

［39］ 朴胜华，郭姣，胡竹平.高脂血症住院患者中医证候临床研究［J］.中国中西医结合杂志，2012，32（10）:1322-1325.

［40］ Ji L,Hu D,Pan C,et al.Primacy of the 3B approach to control risk factors for cardiovascular disease in type 2 diabetes patients［J］.Am J Med,2013,126（10）:925.e11-22.

［41］ 中华医学会肝病学分会脂肪肝和酒精性肝病学组，中国医师协会脂肪性肝病专家委员会.非酒精性脂肪性肝病防治指南（2018年更新版）［J］.实用肝脏病杂志，2018，21（2）:177-186.

［42］ Portillo-Sanchez P,Bril F,Maximos M,et al.High Prevalence of Nonalcoholic Fatty Liver Disease in Patients

With Type 2 Diabetes Mellitus and Normal Plasma Aminotransferase Levels［J］.J Clin Endocrinol Metab,2015,100（6）:2231-2238.

［43］ Leite NC,Villela-Nogueira CA,Pannain VL,et al.Histopathological stages of nonalcoholic fatty liver disease in type 2 diabetes: prevalences and correlated factors［J］.Liver Int,2011,31（5）:700-706.

［44］ Targher G,Bertolini L,Rodella S,et al.Non-alcoholic fatty liver disease is independently associated with an increased prevalence of chronic kidney disease and proliferative/laser-treated retinopathy in type 2 diabetic patients［J］.Diabetologia,2008,51（3）:444-450.

［45］ Zhao Y,Sun H,Wang B,et al.Impaired fasting glucose predicts the development of hypertension over 6 years in female adults: Results from the rural Chinese cohort study［J］.J Diabetes Complications,2017,31（7）:1090-1095.

［46］ Emdin CA,Anderson SG,Woodward M,et al.Usual Blood Pressure and Risk of New-Onset Diabetes: Evidence From 4.1 Million Adults and a Meta-Analysis of Prospective Studies［J］.J Am Coll Cardiol,2015,66（14）:1552-1562.

［47］ Zhang Y,Jiang X,Bo J,et al.Risk of stroke and coronary heart disease among various levels of blood pressure in diabetic and nondiabetic Chinese patients［J］.J Hypertens,2018,36（1）:93-100.

［48］ Pan L,Yang Z,Wu Y,et al.The prevalence,awareness,treatment and control of dyslipidemia among adults in China［J］.Atherosclerosis,2016,248:2-9.

［49］ Pan H,Guo J,Su Z.Advances in understanding the interrelations between leptin resistance and obesity［J］.Physiol Behav,2014,130:157-169.

［50］ 张晶晶.基于HPA轴研究复方贞术调脂方改善糖脂代谢的作用和机制［D］.广州：广东药科大学，2017.

［51］ Ye DW,Rong XL,Xu AM,et al.Liver-adipose tissue crosstalk: A key player in the pathogenesis of glucolipid metabolic disease［J］.Chin J Integr Med,2017,23（6）:410-414.

［52］ Ding C,Guo J,Su Z.The status of research into resistance to diet-induced obesity［J］.Horm Metab Res,2015,47（6）:404-410.

［53］ Saltiel AR,Kahn CR.Insulin signalling and the regulation of glucose and lipid metabolism［J］.Nature,2001,414（6865）:799-806.

［54］ Liu J,Zhuang ZJ,Bian DX,et al.Toll-like receptor-4 signalling in the progression of non-alcoholic fatty liver disease induced by high-fat and high-fructose diet in mice［J］.Clin Exp Pharmacol Physiol,2014,41（7）:482-488.

［55］ Corkey BE.Banting lecture 2011: hyperinsulinemia: cause or consequence［J］.Diabetes, 2012,61（1）:4-13.

［56］ 韦之富.FTZ改善持续炎性反应引起的糖脂代谢紊乱的作用及机制研究［D］.广州：广东药科大学，2017.

［57］ Li M,Han Z,Bei W,et al.Oleanolic Acid Attenuates Insulin Resistance via NF-κB to Regulate the IRS1-GLUT4 Pathway in HepG2 Cells［J］.Evid Based Complement Alternat Med,2015:643102.

［58］ Glass CK,Olefsky JM.Inflammation and lipid signaling in the etiology of insulin resistance［J］.Cell Metab,2012,15（5）:635-645.

［59］ 袁瑜，孙之梅，张扬，等.肠道微生态对非酒精性脂肪性肝病发病与治疗的影响［J］.中华肝脏病杂志，2016，24（5）:375-379.

［60］ Zhong HJ,Yuan Y,Xie WR,et al.Type 2 Diabetes Mellitus Is Associated with More Serious Small Intestinal Mucosal Injuries［J］.PLoS One,2016,11（9）:e0162354.

［61］ 钟豪杰，吴礼浩，陈羽，等.代谢综合征与小肠黏膜损伤的相关性［J］.世界华人消化杂志，2016（11）:1754-1759.

［62］ 鲁媛，罗婷婷，严诗楷，等.代谢组学在高脂血症的研究进展［J］.广东化工，2018，45（10）:133-135.

［63］ 王露莎，寇天顺，黄云翠，等.复方贞术调脂方调节肝脏脂肪酸组成防治非酒精性脂肪肝［J］.世界科学技术 - 中医药现代化，2018，20（5）:734-743.

［64］ 赵慧敏，雷自立，郭姣.脂联素水平与2型糖尿病及心血管疾病矛盾性关系的研究进展［J］.中国细胞生物学学报，2018，40（5）:820-826.

［65］ 刘倩，尹智炜，段姝伟，等.糖尿病肾病中医辨证指南发展及应用［J］.中华肾病研究电子杂志，2018，7（2）:91-93.

［66］ 黄婧文，朴胜华，郭姣.糖脂代谢患者群中医体质类型及舌脉特点分析［J］.中华中医药杂志，2018，33（3）:1082-1084.

［67］ 林育，项磊，肖雪，等.基于临床研究的湿热证文本信息挖掘［J］.广东药科大学学报，2017，33（5）:654-658.

［68］ 张霞，王予娇，曾智桓，等.田黄片对血管内皮损伤后内膜增生的影响［J］.中药新药与临床药理，2017，28（5）:606-610.

［69］ 孙跃，兰天，郭姣.鞘氨醇激酶信号通路在肝纤维化中的作用机制［J］.临床肝胆病杂志，2017，33（9）:1798-1801.

［70］ 付蓉，荣向路，郭姣.复方贞术调脂方对非酒精性脂肪肝的肝PPARα及其下游基因的影响［J］.中国中西医结合杂志，2017，37（6）:735-740.

［71］ 韦之富，雷自立，郭姣.高血糖症的炎性反应机制研究进展［J］.今日药学，2017，27（5）:358-360.

［72］ 李硕，苏诗娜，朴胜华，等.广州市大学生中医体质调查分析［J］.中华中医药杂志,2017,32（4）:1833-1835.

［73］ 张晶晶，蔡金艳，郭姣.11β - 羟基类固醇脱氢酶1在2型糖尿病中的研究进展［J］.食品与药品，2017，19（2）:142-147.

Foreword

The main drafting organizations: Guangdong Pharmaceutical University, Beijing Hospital of Traditional Chinese Medicine affiliated to Capital Medical University, China Academy of Chinese Medical Sciences, Tongji Medical College of Huazhong University of Science and Technology, Affiliated Hospital of Chengdu University of Traditional Chinese Medicine, The First Affiliated Hospital of Anhui University of Traditional Chinese Medicine, The First Affiliated Hospital of Sun Yat-sen University, UniMed Centerl (The United States), Western University (Canada).

The participating organizations: Beijing University of Chinese Medicine, Dongfang Hospital Affiliated to Beijing University of Chinese Medicine, Dongzhimen Hospital Affiliated to Beijing University of Chinese Medicine, Beijing Geriatric Hospital, Chengdu University of TCM, Huashan Hospital Affiliated to Fudan University, Gansu University Of Chinese Medicine, Affiliated Hospital of Gansu University of Traditional Chinese Medicine, The First Affiliated Hospital of Guangdong Pharmaceutical University, Guangzhou Overseas Chinese Hospital, Guangdong Province Hospital of Traditional Chinese Medicine, Guangdong Provincial Association of Chinese Medicine, Guangzhou Medical University, the First Affiliated Hospital of Guangzhou University of Traditional Chinese Medicine, Heilongjiang Traditional Chinese Medicine Hospital, Hunan University of Chinese Medicine, Jilin Provincial Hospital of Traditional Chinese Medicine, School of Traditional Chinese Medicine, Jinan University, The Affiliated Hospital of Jiangxi University of Traditional Chinese Medicine, Liaoning University of Traditional Chinese Medicine, Nanjing University of Chinese Medicine, European Association of Jing Fang TCM (Germany), Shandong Provincial Hospital, Shandong College of Traditional Chinese Medicine, The Affiliated Hospital of Shaanxi University of Chinese Medicine, Cancer Hospital of Shantou University Medical College, Shanghai Institute of Traditional Chinese Medicine, Shanghai Changzheng Hospital , Yueyang Hospital of Integrated Traditional Chinese and Western Medicine ,Shanghai University of Traditional Chinese Medicine, Shanghai University of Traditional Chinese Medicine, Shenzhen Second People's Hospital, Shenzhen Traditional Chinese Medicine Hospital, Tianjin Academy of Traditional Chinese Medicine, Wenzhou Medical University, Yunnan Hospital of Traditional Chinese Medicine, The Second Affiliated Hospital of Zhejiang University school of Medicine, Zhejiang University, Zhejiang Chinese Medical University, Zhengzhou University, Military Academy of Sciences, China Pharmaceutical University, Guang'anmen Hospital, Xiyuan Hospital, Zhongshan Hospital of Traditional Chinese Medicine, ChongQing Medical University, Chinese Medicine and Acupuncture Society of Australia, Belgium Federation of Traditional Chinese Medicine, American Allegiant Health Company ,A&Z Pharmaceutical Inc(The United States), Texas Health And Science University, The Integrated Medical Center of Vanderbilt University(The United States), St. John's UniMed(The United States), The University of Hong Kong, HKU Li Ka Shing Faculty of Medicine,The Hong Kong University of Science and Technology, The Chinese University of Hong Kong, The Hong Kong Yongkang Pharmaceutical Limited company.

The main drafters of this standard: Jiao Guo, Shengsheng Zhang, Yan Lei, Fuer Lu, Chunguang Xie, Zhaohui Fang, Jun Tao, Haoyi Liu (The United States), Subrata Chakrabarti (Canada).

Drafting participants and review experts (in alphabetical order of the last name):

China: Xiaodong Bie, Weiguo Cao, Zhuhong Chen, Fuchun Cheng, Yihui Deng, Yuhong Duan, Guanjie Fan,Nanlin Fu, Zhongnong Fan, Yue Gao, Sihua Gao, Yanbing Gong,Xingxiang He, Yiyang Hu, Zhenshan Jiao, Ling Jin, Shiming Jin, Xuedong Kang, Haixue Kuang, Guobiao Li, Huilin Li, Leyu Li, Xianzhu Li, Yingdong Li, Zhongwei Lin,Jianpin Liu, Yi Liu, Zhongyong Liu, Guoan Luo, Yi Ma, Chunli Piao, Shenghua Piao, Xianglu Rong, Dazhuo Shi, Zongliang Song, Huilin Sun, Xiaolin Tong, Haitong Wan, Jianwei Wang, Junping Wei, Bo Wen, Jun Wu, Yiling Wu, Zonggui Wu, Xiang Lei, Wenhao Xia, Xia Xu, Haibo Xu, Yanqiu Xu, Zhen Yang, Jiehong Yang, Xiaohui Yang, Yufeng Yang, Wenbing Yao, Dewei Ye, Qiuxia Yi, Ling Yi, Xintong Yu, Xiyong Yu, Zhihuan Zeng, Libin Zhan, Zhou Qiang, Teng Zhang, Guangde Zhang, Jianyong Zhang, Qinghua Zhang, Shuyao Zhang, Wanxing Zhou, Zhangzhi Zhu.

Hong Kong, China: Yibin Feng, Huangquan Lin, Yi Niu, Shiming Ni, Aimin Xu, Cuifeng Zhu.

The United States: Zhesheng Chen, Yuxin He, Zihong Li, Haoyi Liu, Chongbing Zhu.

Australia: Yuhao Li, Jianhua Zheng.

Belgium: Lilin Tao.

Canada: Subrata Chakrabarti.

Germany: Feng Li.

The drafting procedures of this standard were consistent with SCM 0001-2009 *Working Regulation for Formu1ation and Publication of Standard* and document of *2011 (No. 20) Implementation of Technical Standards of the Specialized Committee* released by World Federation of Chinese Medicine Societies (WFCMS).

Introduction

The glucolipid metabolism diseases refer to a patient with dyslipidemia, nonalcoholic fatty liver disease(NAFLD), obesity, hypertension, atherosclerotic cardiovascular disease, Cardio-cerebrovascular disease etc. Its high incidence is a worldwide crisis.

According to IDF Diabetes Atlas (8th edition) released by International Diabetes Federation (IDF), some 425 million people worldwide, or 8.8% of adults 20~79 years, are estimated to have diabetes while 114 million adults with diabetes (20~79 years) in China account for 10.9%. In addition, the prevalence of dyslipidemia, NAFLD, obesity, hypertension and other diseases stays high and is rising year by year, bringing great threaten to human health.

In recent years, epidemiological studies have gradually focused on the harm of complications and compound diseases in glucolipid metabolism diseases. In 2008, Professor Guo Jiao's led a team to first investigate the morbidity of hyperlipidemia patients, and the results showed that 84.2% of hyperlipidemia patients had the complication of hyperglycemia and hypertension and other diseases. From 2010 to 2012, a "3B" study found out that 72% of T2DM patients are associated with hypertension and/or dyslipidemia. Compared with patients with T2DM alone, patients with T2DM combined with dyslipidemia and hypertension had six times higher risk in having cardiovascular disease. Moreover, studies also confirmed that diabetes mellitus, dyslipidemia and nonalcoholic fatty liver disease can significantly increase the risk of microvascular and macrovascular complications in patients with diabetes.

The above results show that pathoglycemia, dyslipidemia, hypertension and nonalcoholic fatty liver disease are often closely related, mutually complicated and interactively influenced. Currently, single disease-targeted therapy is adopted for the diagnosis and treatment for Glucolipid Metabolic Disorders, but the control on dyslipidemia and hypertension is relatively low. Therefore, comprehensive understanding and prevention and control on Glucolipid Metabolic Disorders are needed to improve the effectiveness.

Under such condition, Professor Guo Jiao in Guangdong Pharmaceutical University first put forward the concept of "Glucolipid Metabolic Disorders(Dan-Zhuo)" and it was widely recognized both in China and abroad. In 2015, the Lingnan International Forum on Metabolic Diseases reached a "Guangdong Consensus" on Glucolipid Metabolic Disorders. In view of the lack of relevant standard, this standard is hereby formulated to further standardize the clinical diagnosis and treatment of Glucolipid Metabolic Disorders and provide Chinese and Western medicine treatment strategies and methods for clinical practice.

Specification of Diagnosis and Treatment of Glucolipid Metabolic Disorders (Dan-Zhuo) with Integrated Chinese and Western Medicine

1 Scope

The standard specifies the definition, etiology and pathogenesis, criteria for the diagnosis, syndrome differentiation and treatment for Glucolipid Metabolic Disorders (Dan-Zhuo).

This standard applies to medical and scientific research institutions engaged in clinical diagnosis, treatment and scientific research of Glucolipid Metabolic Disorders (Dan-Zhuo) at various levels.

2 Normative References

There are no normative references in this document.

3 Terms and Definitions

The following terms and definitions apply to this document.

3.1

Glucolipid Metabolic Disorders

Glucolipid Metabolic Disorders diseases characterized by the disorders of glucolipid metabolism and resulted from a variety of factors involving genetics, environment, spirit, and diet, with neuroendocrine dysfunction, insulin resistance, oxidative stress, chronic inflammation and intestinal flora imbalanced as the core pathologies, associated with single hyperglycemia, lipid disorders, fatty liver, obesity, hypertension, atherosclerosis etc. or several as the main clinical manifestations, which require a comprehensive prevention and control.

Note: It belongs to "Dan-Zhuo" in TCM.

3.2

"Dan-Zhuo" Disease

"Dan-Zhuo" Disease characterized by mood depression or impatience, body fat or thin, head and body sleepy heavy, bitter taste and sticky sensation in mouth, fullness and discomfort or pain in chest and hypochondrium, fatigue and lack of strength, dry throat and mouth as the main clinical manifestations, with dampness retention, phlegm turbidity, stasis, heat evil as its main pathogenic factors and dysfunction of the liver in dispersing as its main pathogenesis playing a key role in disease progress and prognosis, caused by emotional disorders, improper diet, constitutional deficiency, old age and feeble body condition.

Note: "Dan" mainly refers to heat, damp-heat or consumptive disease and it may lead to the damage of many organs, including spleen, stomach, kidney, heart, liver, gallbladder, etc.;"Zhuo" refers to dampness, phlegm, stasis, heat, and other pathological turbidity. In modern medicine, the pathological changes and products of glucose and lipid metabolism disorders, including hyperglycemia, hyperlipidemia, nonalcoholic fatty liver, overweight, hypertension, and atherosclerotic plaques all belong to "Dan-Zhuo".

4 Pathogenesis

4.1 Pathogenesis from Western Medicine

4.1.1 Neurological - Endocrine - Immune disorder

Specific neurons in the brain can perceive the changes in metabolic substrates; meanwhile, it is able to interact with leptin, insulin and other cytokines through the blood-brain barrier to regulate the metabolism of glucose and lipid in vivo.

4.1.2 Insulin Resistance

Insulin resistance plays a key role in the metabolism disorder of both glucose and lipid. If the insulin signal pathway of liver, fat, muscle, brain and other effector organs is blocked, the insulin sensitivity may decline, leading to systemic glucose and lipid metabolism disorders.

4.1.3 Oxidative Stress

Oxidative stress is a vital basis for abnormal glucose and lipid metabolism. Both glucose and lipid toxicity can damage islet cells, muscle, fat cell and insulin receptors through oxidative stress, thus causing insulin resistance. At the same time, it damages vascular endothelial cells, leading to extensive cardiovascular and cerebrovascular diseases.

4.1.4 Chronic Inflammation

Chronic inflammation is common in the pathogenesis of abnormal glucolipid metabolism. Inflammatory signaling molecules are involved in regulating metabolic organs, such as liver, fat, muscle, pancreas and other glucose and lipid metabolism through the widely interwoven immune network. The anti-inflammatory treatment of GLMD is also a key focus of current research.

4.1.5 The Imbalance of the Intestinal Flora

Intestinal flora plays an important role in glucose and lipid metabolism in the body. Intestinal flora may affect glucose and lipid metabolism by regulating inflammatory reaction and controlling immune system. Therefore, the disorders of the intestinal flora may lead to obesity, hyperlipidemia, diabetes, atherosclerosis and other metabolic disorders.

4.2 Etiology and Pathogenesis from Chinese Medicine

4.2.1 Etiology

Emotional disorders; improper diet, or favor to oily, greasy and fatty food; constitutional deficiency, or feeble body condition due to old age, or overwork, or too much sexual intercourse.

4.2.2 Disease Location

The disease mainly involves the liver, spleen and kidney, and the heart, brain and viscera veins are affected in the later stage.

4.2.3 Pathogenesis

The dysfunction of the liver in dispersing results in that the five Zang-organs and six Fu-organs are all involved and disturbed, leading to the disorder of transportation of essence of water and grain and body fluid and fat accumulation, and turning into "Dan" after a long period or forming dampness, phlegm, blood stasis, poison and other turbid. "Dan" and "Zhuo" interact and finally become "Dan-Zhuo". The dysfunction of the liver in dispersing is the main pathogenesis, playing a key role in disease progress and prognosis. Dampness, phlegm, stasis, heat and toxin are the main pathological products.

The liver controls the dispersion and regulates emotions, including adjusting one's emotions, assisting spleen and stomach to transport and transform, and promoting the transportation of blood and fluid. The long-term pressure and anxiety may cause uneasiness in emotion, and then the liver qi will be depressed and stagnated and later restrict the spleen. The improper diet, longing forgreasy or fatty food or too much thinking can all impair the spleen and stomach, leading to the deficiency. The dysfunction of the spleen in transportation leads to internal generation of phlegm and dampness for the poor digestion, which will gradually generate stagnant heat and even toxic heat. Meanwhile, the liver qi depression will cause qi stagnation and blood stasis or qi stagnation and phlegm coagulation, and even the obstruction of phlegm and blood stasis after a rather long time. Moreover, qi depression will transform into fire, and fire-heat and phlegm-heat impair qi and yin, causing deficiency of both qi and yin. The constitutional deficiency, feeble body condition due to the old age, overwork or too much sexual intercourse and the spleen diseases affecting the kidney may all result in the failure in steaming body fluid into qi due to damage to deficiency of kidney yang. The depression and stagnation of liver qi and the disturbance of blood and fluid transportation may bring out water toxin inundation and internal obstruction of stasis turbidity.Consequently, the disease is caused by the imbalance of transportation and distribution of the qi, blood and body fluid, thus leading to the accumulation of dampness, phlegm, stasis, heat and other turbidity. In the late stage, the kidney essence is insufficient, unable to warm and nourish the five zang-organs and six fu-organs, while the dampness, phlegm, stasis, heat and toxicity then accumulate and blockage and damage of the collaterals are more serious. Finally, multiple pathological factors coexist, corresponding viscera and fu-organs are affected, deficiency and excess in complexity aggravate the disease and then it takes longer time to treat and hard to heal.

5 Diagnosis from Western Medicine

According to the pathological process, Glucolipid Metabolic Disorders can be divided into three stages. There are no clinical symptoms in stage I , only mild changes in blood biochemical indicators and/or imaging indexes; corresponding clinical symptoms in stage II , the changes of blood biochemical indicators and/or images reach the clinical diagnostic criteria; in stage III , the condition worsen on the basis of stage II , and there are complications.

5.1 Stage I of Glucolipid Metabolic Disorders

The diagnosis of stage I of Glucolipid Metabolic Disorders shall meet the criteria in Appendix A, as well as one or more of the following three indicators.

a) Pre-diabetes.

b) The blood lipids is normal but at the margin, with two or more risk factors.

    1) Obesity BMI ≥ 28 kg/m^2.

    2) Smoking ≥ 1 year, ≥ 1 per day.

    3) Those with inherited or familial hyperlipidemia.

    4) Family history [i] of early onset atherosclerotic vascular disease [ii].

Note: i: Refers to male relatives of the immediate family before the age of 55 or female direct relatives before the age of 65 with ischemic cardiovascular disease. ii: Carotid stenosis $\geq 50\%$, renal artery stenosis $\geq 50\%$, arteriosclerosis occlusive disease of lower extremities, coronary heart disease, cerebral infarction.

c) Nonalcoholic fatty liver disease.

5.2 Stage Ⅱ of Glucolipid Metabolic Disorders

The diagnosis of stage Ⅱ of Glucolipid Metabolic Disorders shall meet the criteria of Appendix B and any one or more of the following 4 indicators shall be met.

a) Type 2 diabetes.

b) Abnormal blood lipids.

c) Nonalcoholic steatohepatitis (NASH).

d) Carotid or other atherosclerotic plaques, but stenosis<50%.

5.3 Stage Ⅲ of Glucolipid Metabolic Disorders

The diagnosis of stage III of Glucolipid Metabolic Disorders shall meet the criteria of Appendix C, and any one or more of the following 3 indicators shall be met.

a) Diabetes with chronic complications.

b) Atherosclerotic vascular disease (carotid stenosis ≥ 50%, renal artery stenosis ≥ 50%, arteriosclerosis occlusive disease of lower extremities, coronary heart disease, cerebral infarction) on the basis of stage II of glucolipid metabolism.

c) Nonalcoholic fatty liver fibrosis or cirrhosis.

6 Diagnostic Syndrome Criteria from Chinese Medicine

The disease can be classified into the following seven syndrome types. The syndrome of liver stagnation and spleen deficiency is common in Glucolipid Metabolic Disorders stage Ⅰ; the syndrome of phlegm obstruction, syndrome of dampness-heat, and syndrome of qi and yin deficiency are common in the stage Ⅱ; spleen-kidney yang deficiency syndrome, Phlegm-Stasis accumulation syndrome, yang deficiency and turbidity syndrome are common in stage Ⅲ.

6.1 Syndrome of Liver Stagnation and Spleen Deficiency

Depression with frequent sighing, fatigue, distention or scurrying pain in the chest and flank, anorexia, abdominal distention, borborigmus with flatus, loose stool, pale scalloped tongue, white and thin coating, and stringy or stringy-thready pulse.

6.2 Syndrome of Phlegm Obstruction

The subjective sensation of heaviness in the head and body, pectoral and abdominal stuffiness, nausea, expectoration of phlegm, sticky and greasy sensation in the mouth, anorexia, overweight or obesity, light tongue, enlarged or scalloped tongue body with white and thick coating, and slippery or soggy pulse.

6.3 Syndrome of Dampness-Heat

Gastric stuffiness, greasy face, bitter taste, red eyes with discharge, anorexia and poor appetite, heavy cumbersome limbs, dull fever, yellowish urine, sticky and foul stool, red tongue, yellow and greasy coating, slippery and rapid pulse.

6.4 Syndrome of Qi and Yin Deficiency

Lack of strength and shortness of breath, aggravated after exercise, dry mouth, pale face with lack of luster or flushed cheek, heat in the palms and soles, insomnia and dreaminess, spontaneous and night sweating, constipation, red tongue with scant liquid, thin white or scant coating, and thready or feeble pulse.

6.5 Syndrome of Spleen-Kidney Yang Deficiency

Cold limbs, waist, knees and abdomen, pale face, edema of face and limbs, palpitation, frequent nocturia, loose stool or undigested food in stool, frequent defecation or diarrhea before dawn, pale tongue, enlarged and teeth-marked tongue body with white and slippery coating, and deep, thready, slow pulse or feeble, slow pulse.

6.6 Syndrome of Phlegm-Stasis Accumulation

Stuffy pain or stabbing pain in chest, dark and lusterless face, chest oppression and gastric stuffiness, cough and phlegm, dizziness or headache, aphasia, limb numbness or pain, or even hemiplegia, darkish tongue or with stasis speckles or maculae on the sides, white or greasy coating, stringy and slippery or deep and unsmooth pulse.

6.7 Syndrome of Yang Deficiency and Turbidity

Mental fatigue and somnolence, cold limbs or even whole body swelling, darkish complexion, dementia in mind, cough and panting with phlegm, suffocation with short breath, nausea or vomiting, drum-like abdominal distention, soreness and weakness of waist and knees, itching in the itching in the skin, wilted limbs and foot carbuncle, short voiding with scant urine, pale tongue with teeth marks on sides, turbid and greasy coating, deep slow and feeble pulse.

7 Treatment Target and Principles

7.1 Treatment Target

Comprehensive prevention and treatment from the perspectives of Western medicine pathogenesis and TCM etiology and pathogenesis shall be carried out, to reduce or delay the occurrence of chronic complications, and improve the effectiveness in prevention and control of Glucolipid Metabolic Disorders and its clinical recovery.

7.2 Western Medicine Treatment

7.2.1 Treatment for Stage I of Glucolipid Metabolic Disorders is mainly for therapeutic lifestyle changes (TLC).

a) Healthy diet, daily intake of carbohydrates (mainly vegetables, fruits, beans, whole grains et al.) accounting for 50% to 65% of the total energy are recommended; the intake of fat shall not exceed 20% to 30% of the total energy, and the saturated fatty acid intake shall be less than 7% of the total energy, and the trans fatty acid intake shall be Less than 1% of total energy. Foods with higher fiber and lower sugar load are recommended. Mediterranean diets rich in monounsaturated and polyunsaturated fatty acids are recommended.

b) Regular exercise, 5~7 times a week, 30-minute exercise of moderate intensity.

c) Quitting smoking completely and effectively avoiding inhaling second-hand smoke and restricting alcohol consumption.

d) Maintaining optimal body weight with BMI between 20.0~23.9 kg/m^2. Women aged over 60 with BMI>35 kg/m^2 and a history of hyperglycemia in pregnancy, are advised to use metformin to prevent type 2 diabetes.

7.2.2 Treatment for Stage II of Glucolipid Metabolic Disorders, on the basis of the TLC, according to the individual's risk to arteriosclerotic cardiovascular disease (ASCVD) and the patient's blood sugar, is mainly by lipid regulation, sugar-reducing, anti-inflammation and liver protection.

a) Lipid regulation is to reduce LDL-C levels as the primary intervention strategy to prevent ASCVD risk. The target values for lipid-lowering therapy are as follows: LDL-C<1.8 mmol/L for extreme high-risk patients; LDL-C<2.6 mmol/L for high-risk patients; LDL-C<3.4 mmol/L for intermediate-risk and low-risk patients. If the LDL-C baseline value is too high to reach the target value, LDL-C shall be reduced by at least 50%. For very high-risk patients, if the LDL-C baseline is within the target value, it shall still be reduced by about 30%. According to the patient's condition, the corresponding drugs are selected. For hypercholesterolemia and mixed hyperlipidemia, statins represented by atorvastatin are preferred, and if statins can not meet the standard, it can be combined with cholesterol absorption inhibitors, such as ezetimibe; for hypertriglyceridemia, with TG $\geq$ 5.7 mmol / L, fibrates, such as fenofibrate, are preferred; niacin or high purity fish oil formulations can reduce triglyceride as well.

b) Sugar-reducing, blood sugar control refers to the American Diabetes Association (2018) (Figure 1, Figure 2).

At diagnosis, initiate lifestyle management, set A1C target, and initiate pharmacologic therapy based on A1C

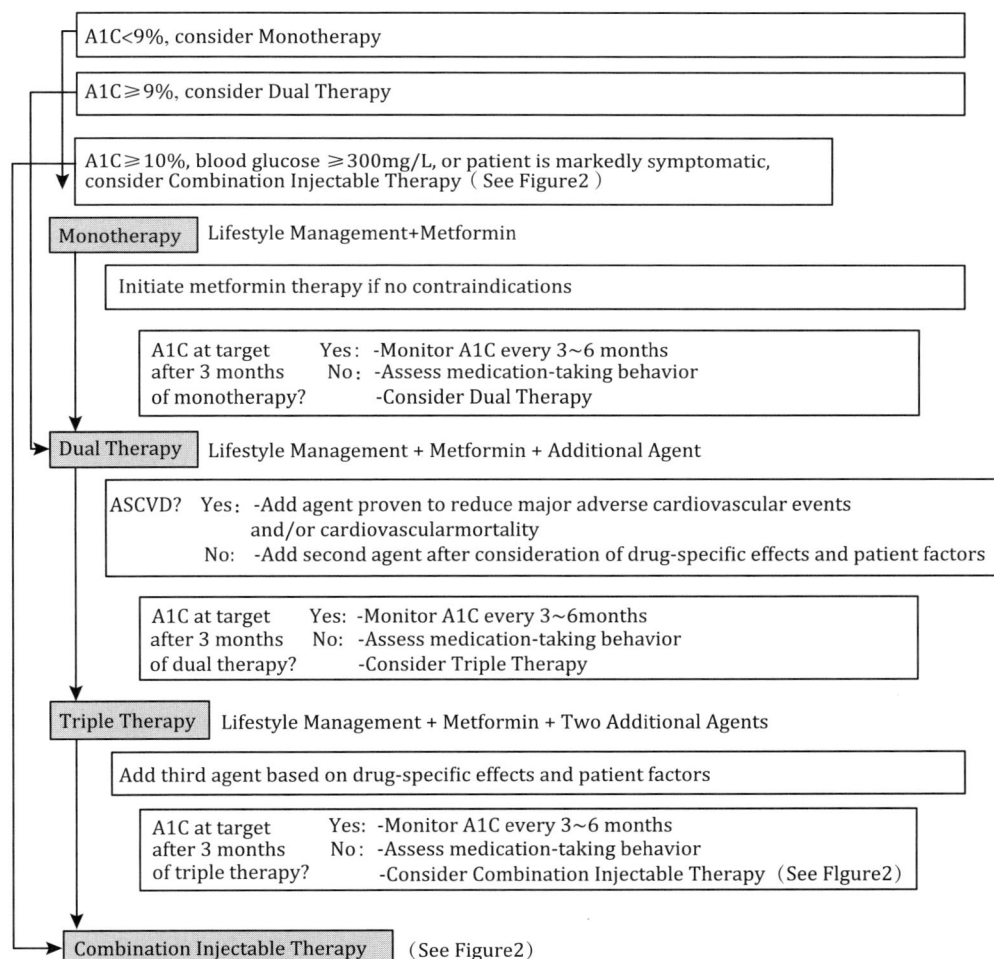

Figure 1   Treatment Principles for blood sugar control

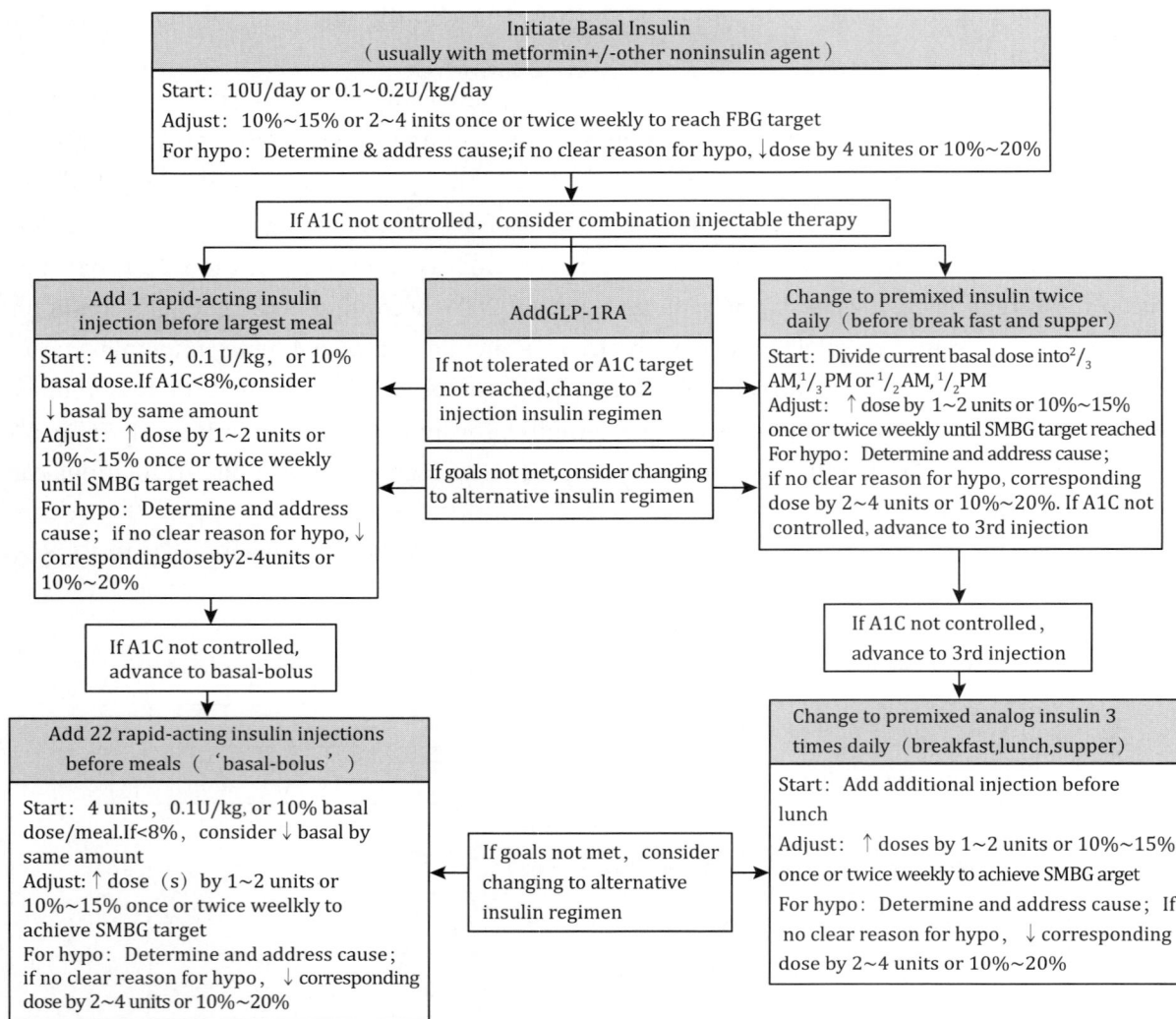

Figure 2　Combination therapy for blood glucose control

c) Anti-inflammatory and liver protection, patients with nonalcoholic steatohepatitis, add anti-inflammatory and liver-protecting drugs, such as bicyclol,Magnesium Isoglycyrrhizinate injection, etc., while supplementing probiotics, and bacterial transplantation treatment may also be considered.

7.2.3 Stage Ⅲ of Glucolipid Metabolic Disorders, corresponding treatment for complications.

a) For those who do not meet the standard with treatment of statin alone, the combination of cholesterol absorption inhibitors and statin shall be recommended. For those still with poor efficacy may choose a novel lipid-lowering drug proprotein convertase subtilisin/kexin type9 (PSCK9) inhibitor, such as Alirocumab; and on the basis of individualized lipid-lowering, strictly control other high-risk factors by the use of aspirin, clopidogrel and other antiplatelet drugs to prevent complications.

b) Patients with severe stenosis or even occlusion of the target arteries shall be treated with appropriate thrombolysis, balloon dilatation or stent implantation.

c) For the chronic complications of diabetes or non-alcoholic fatty liver cirrhosis, the corresponding symptomatic treatment shall be carried out on the basis of correcting the disorder of glucose and lipid metabolism.

7.3 TCM Treatment

The stage Ⅰ of Glucolipid Metabolic Disorders is mainly caused by liver stagnation and spleen deficiency. It can be treated by soothing liver to regulate the emotions and regulating the ascending and descending of qi movement, and invigorating spleen to eliminate turbid, strengthen the ability to regulate qi, blood and body fluids, and maintain metabolic balance. The stage Ⅱ of Glucolipid Metabolic Disorders commonly shows as deficiency-excess in complexity. Deficiency syndrome mainly manifests as qi and yin deficiency, treated by replenishing qi and nourishing yin; excess syndrome is mainly caused by dampness, phlegm, and heat accumulation in body, treated by regulating liver to smooth qi movement, opening the hub to motivate transportation and transformation, and clearing heat, eliminating dampness and resolving phlegm to maintain the movement of qi, blood, and body fluid and regulate turbidity metabolism. The stage Ⅲ of Glucolipid Metabolic Disorders still shows as deficiency-excess in complexity mostly. Deficiency syndrome mainly manifests as spleen-kidney yang deficiency, treated by warming and tonifying spleen and kidney; excess syndrome is dominated by phlegm-stasis accumulation syndrome with yang deficiency, turbidity and toxin, vessels and networks damage, treated by dispelling stasis and resolving phlegm, eliminating turbidity and removing toxin. Meanwhile, if serious patients have the decline of brain, heart and kidney, they shall be mainly treated by zang-fu organs differentiation.

7.3.1 Syndrome of Liver Stagnation and Spleen Deficiency

Therapeutic Method: Soothing liver and invigorating spleen.

Prescription: Modified Xiaoyao Powder (*Preions of the Bureau of Taiping People's Welfare Pharmacy*).

Ingredients: Chaihu (Radix Bupleuri), Danggui (Radix Angelicae Sinensis), Baishao (Radix Paeoniae Alba), Baizhu (Rhizoma Atractylodis Macrocephalae), Fuling (Poria), roasting Shengjiang (Rhizoma Zingiberis), Bohe (Herba Menthae) and stir-frying with liquid adjuvant Gancao (Radix Glycyrrhizae).

Addition and subtraction: If a patient combined with severe hypochondriac pain, Danshen (Radix Salviae Miltiorrhizae), Qingpi (Vatica Mangachapoi Blauco), Yujin (Radix Curcumae), Foshou (Fructus Citri Sarcodactylis) shall be added. If combined with severe abdominal distension, Houpo (Magnolia officinalis Rehd. et Wils.), Muxiang (Aucklandiae Radix) shall be added. If combined with severe loose stool, Shanyao (Rhizoma Dioscoreae), Dangshen (Radix Codonopsis), Sharen (Fructus Amomi Villosi) shall be added. If combined with vexation and anger, Danpi (Moutan Cortex), stir-frying Zhizi (Gardenia jasminoides Ellis), Nvzhenzi (Fructus Ligustri Lucidi) shall be added.

7.3.2 Syndrome of Phlegm Obstruction

Therapeutic Method: regulating qi and resolving phlegm and eliminating dampness.

Prescription: Modified Erchen Decoction and Pingwei Powder (Preions of the Bureau of Taiping People's Welfare Pharmacy).

Ingredients: Erchen Decoction: processed Banxia (Rhizoma Pinelliae)with Ginger, Chenpi (Pericarpium Citri Reticulatae), Fuling (Poria), stir-frying Gancao (Radix Glycyrrhizae).

Pingwei Powder: Cangzhu (Atractylodes Rhizome), Houpo (Cortex Magnoliae Officinalis), Jupi (Pericarpium Citri Reticulatae), Gancao (Radix Glycyrrhizae), Shengjiang (Rhizoma Zingiberis) and Dazao (Ziziphus jujuba Mill).

Addition and subtraction: If combined with severe stuffiness and fullness in chest and hypochondrium, Zhiqiao (Citrus aurantium), Gualou (Trichosanthes kirilowii Maxim), Xiebai (Allium macrostemon Bunge) shall be added. If combined with phlegm rale in the throat, Dannanxing (Rhizoma Arisaematis Cum Bile), Suzi (Perillafrutescens) shall be added. If combined with obvious dizziness, Gouteng (Ramulus Uncariae cum Uncis) Tianma (Gastrodia elata Bl.), Baizhu (Atractylodes macrocephala) shall be added. If combined with insomnia, Yejiaoteng (Caulis Polygoni Multiflori), Yuanzhi (Polygala tenuifolia Willd), Dannanxing (Rhizoma Arisaematis Cum Bile), Shichangpu (Rhizoma Acori Tatarinowii), Fushen (（Poria cocos Schw.）Wolf) shall be added.

7.3.3　Syndrome of Dampness-Heat

Therapeutic Method: clearing heat and resolving dampness.

Prescription: a) If the dampness-heat is accumulated in the middle energizer, Lianpo Decoction (*Cholera theory*) shall be chosen.

b) If the dampness-heat is accumulated in the lower energizer, Modified Gegen Huangqin Huanglian Decoction (*Treatise on Cold Damage Diseases*) or Simiao Pill (*A Convenient Reading for Precription*) shall be chosen.

Ingredients: Lianpo Decoction, Houpo (Cortex Magnoliae Officinalis), Huanglian (Rhizoma Coptidis), Shichangpu (Rhizoma Acori Tatarinowii), processed Banxia (Rhizoma Pinelliae), Dandouchi (Semen Sojae Praeparatum), stir-frying Zhizi (Gardenia jasminoides Ellis) to brown, Lugen (Rhizoma Phragmitis). Gegen Huangqin Huanglian Decoction, Gegen (Radix Puerariae), Huangqin (Radix Scutellariae), Huanglian (Rhizoma Coptidis) and Gancao (Radix Glycyrrhizae). Simiao Pill, Chuanhuangbai (Phellodendron chinense Schneid), Yiyiren (Semen Coicis), Cangzhu (Atractylodes Rhizome), Huainiuxi (Achyranthes bidentata Blume).

Addition and subtraction: If combined with anorexia, Shenqu (Massa Medicata Fermentata), Lianqiao (Forsythia suspensa) and Jineijin (Galli Gigeriae Endothelium Corneum) shall be added. If combined with bitter taste in mouth, Chaihu (Radix Bupleuri), Yujin (Radix Curcumae) and Yinchen (Artemisiacapillaris Thunb) shall be added. If presented as red eyes with discharges, Longdancao (Gentiana scabra Bunge) and Xiakucao (Prunella vulgaris L) shall be added. If combined with yellowish urine, Zexie (Rhizoma Alismatis), Daji (Herba Cirsii Japonici), Cheqianzi (Semen Plantaginis) shall be added.

7.3.4　Syndrome of Qi and Yin Deficiency

Therapeutic Method: replenishing qi and nourishing yin.

Prescription: Modified Shenqi Dihuang Decoction (Treasure of syndrome differentiation).

Ingredients: Renshen (Ginseng), Huangqi (Astragali Radix), prepared Dihuang (Radix Rehmanniae Preparata), Fuling (Poria), Shanyao (Dioscorea opposita), Mudanpi (Moutan Cortex), Shanzhuyyu (Cornus officinalis Sieb. et Zucc).

Addition and subtraction: If patients feel thirst with desire to drink a lot, Tianhuafen (Radix Trichosanthis), Shengdihuang (Radix Rehmanniae Recens) and Yuzhu (Polygonatum odoratum（Mill.）Druce) shall be added. If combined with spontaneous and night sweating, Fuxiaomai (Fructus Tritici Levis), calcining Longgu (Os Draconis), calcining Muli (Concha Ostreae) and Wuweizi (Fructus Schisandrae Chinensis) shall be added. If combined with constipation, Baiziren (Semen Platycladi), Huomaren (Fructus Cannabis) and Maidong (Radix Ophiopogonis) shall be added. If combined with dizziness, Gouteng (Ramulus Uncariae cum Uncis), Tianma (Rhizoma Gastrodiae) and Banxia (Rhizoma Pinelliae) shall be added. If combined with severe tinnitus, Shichangpu (Rhizoma Acori Tatarinowii),

Huainiuxi (Achyranthes bidentata Blume) and Duzhong (Eucommia ulmoides) shall be added. If combined with insomnia, stir-frying Suanzaoren (Semen Ziziphi Spinosae) and Baiziren (Semen Platycladi) shall be added.

7.3.5 Syndrome of Spleen-Kidney Yang Deficiency

Therapeutic Method: warming and tonifying spleen and kidney.

Prescription: Modified Fuzi Lizhong Pill (*Preions of the Bureau of Taiping People's Welfare Pharmacy*) and Zhenwu Decoction (*Treatise on Cold Damage*).

Ingredients: Fuzi Lizhong Pill: processed Fuzi (Radix Aconiti Lateralis Preparata Common Monkshood Daughter Root), Renshen (Ginseng), Ganjiang (Dried Ginger), stir-frying Gancao (Radix Glycyrrhizae), Baizhu (White Atractylodes Rhizome).

Zhenwu Decoction: processed Fuzi (Radix Aconiti Lateralis Preparata Common Monkshood Daughter Root), Baizhu (White Atractylodes Rhizome), Shengjiang (Rhizoma Zingiberis), Fuling (Poria) and Shaoyao (Radix Paeoniae).

Addition and subtraction: If combined with palpitation, Rougui (Cortex Cinnamomi), Gejie (Gekko gecko) and Wuweizi (Fructus Schisandrae Chinensis) shall be added. If combined with frequent urination at night, Duzhong (Cortex Eucommiae), Jinyingzi (Cherokee Rose Fruit) and Qianshi (Gordon Euryale Seed) shall be added. If combined with chronic diarrhea or diarrhea before dawn, Wuzhuyu (Medicinal Evodia Fruit), Roudoukou (Semen Myristicae) and Buguzhi (Psoralea corylifolia Linn) shall be added. If combined with edema, Guizhi (Ramulus Cinnamomi), Zexie (Rhizoma Alismatis), Zhuling (Polyporus) and Dafupi (Areca Seed Semen Arecae) shall be added.

7.3.6 Syndrome of Phlegm-Stasis Accumulation

Therapeutic Method: resolving phlegm and dispelling stasis.

Prescription: Modified Gualou Xiebai Banxia Decoction (*Synopsis of the Golden Chamber*) and Xuefu Zhuyu Decoction (*Correction of Errors inMedical Classics*).

Ingredients: Xuefu Zhuyu Decoction: Taoren (Semen Persicae), Honghua (Safflower), Danggui (Radix Angelicae Sinensis), Shengdihuang (Radix Rehmanniae) is added), Niuxi (Achyranthes bidentata Blume), Chuanxiong (Sichuan Lovage Rhizome), Jiegeng (Platycodon grandiflorus), Chishao (Radix Paeoniae Rubra), Zhiqiao (Citrus aurantium), Gancao (Radix Glycyrrhizae) and Chaihu (Radix Bupleuri).

Gualou Xiebai Banxia Decoction: Gualou (Trichosanthes kirilowii Maxim), Xiebai (Allium macrostemon Bunge), Banxia (Rhizoma Pinelliae) and alcohol.

Addition and subtraction: If combined with severe numbness and pain in limbs, Sanqi (Radix et Rhizoma Notoginseng), Jixueteng (Kadsurae Caulis), Guizhi (Ramulus Cinnamomi) and Dilong (Pheretima) shall be added. If combined with phlegm rale in throat, Shichangpu (Rhizoma Acori Tatarinowii), Juhong (Exocarpium Citri Grandis) and Zhebeimu (Bulbus Fritillariae) shall be added. If combined with abdominal distention, Zhishi (Fructus Aurantii Immaturus), Houpo (Cortex Magnoliae Officinalis) shall be added. If combined with severe headache, Dilong (Pheretima), Quanxie (Buthus martensi Karsch) and Xixin (Manchurian Wildginger) shall be added.

7.3.7 Syndrome of Yang Deficiency and Turbidity

Therapeutic Method: warming yang and eliminating turbidity.

Prescription: Modified Wenpi Decoction (A Thousand Gold Pieces Prescriptions).

Ingredients: Fuzi (Radix Aconiti Lateralis Preparata Common Monkshood Daughter Root),

Dahuang (Radix et Rhizoma Rhei), Danggui (Radix Angelicae Sinensis), Ganjiang (Dried Ginger), Renshen (Ginseng) and Gancao (Radix Glycyrrhizae).

Addition and subtraction: If combined with severe suffocation and short breath, stir-frying Mahuang (Ephedra sinica Stapf), Xingren (Semen Armeniacae Amarum), Danshen (Salvia miltiorrhiza Bunge) and Sanqi (Panax notoginseng) shall be added. If combined with severe vomiting, Wuzhuyu (Tetradium ruticarpum), Huanglian (Rhizoma Coptidis) and Shengjiang (Ginger) shall be added. If combined with itching in the skin, Shetui (Elaphe carinata), Danggui (Radix Angelicae Sinensis), Difuzi (Fructus Kochiae) and Baixianpi (Cortex Dictamni) for external use shall be added. If combined with short and scant urine, Guizhi (Ramulus Cinnamomi), Zexie (Rhizoma Alismatis) and Fuling (Poria) shall be added.

For patients in this period are severe and to the advantages in the treatment of Chinese medicine and western medicine should be fully carried out. If necessary, the methods of protecting the liver, strengthening the heart and protecting the kidney should be adopted aiming at the dysfunction of corresponding organs.

8 Comprehensive prevention and control measures

In addition to the above-mentioned Chinese and Western medicine treatment, the Glucolipid Metabolic Disorders can also be treated with acupuncture, warm compress, Tuina, etc. Patients shall pay attention to diet control, exercise, weight loss and other health control methods at the same time, supplemented by psychological adjustment etc to comprehensively control the incidence and further progress of Glucolipid Metabolic Disorders.

APPENDIX A
(Normative Appendix)
Diagnostic Methods for Stage Ⅰ of GLMD

A.1 Diagnostic Criteria for Pre-diabetes (IGT/IFG)

Referred to *WHO Diabetes Diagnostic Criteria, 1999.*

Before the onset of diabetes, there is a period of insulin resistance and islet β-cell damage, called prediabetes. Impaired Fasting Hyperglycemia (IFG) is a state of higher than normal fasting blood (or plasma) glucose concentration, but is lower than the diagnostic cut-off for diabetes.

Impaired Glucose Tolerance (IGT) is a state of higher than normal blood (or plasma) glucose concentration 2 hours after 75 gram oral glucose load but less than the diagnostic cut-off for diabetes At this time, blood glucose levels are higher than normal, but have not yet reached the current diagnostic criteria for diabetes, also known as impaired glucose regulation (IGR). According to fasting and post-load blood glucose values, IGR can be divided into two types of hyperglycemia: impaired fasting glucose (IFG) and impaired glucose tolerance (IGT).

Table A.1　Prediabetes Classification-1999, WHO

	Fasting Glucose（mmol/L）	Glucose of 2h after Meal（mmol/L）
Impaired Fasting Glucose（IFG）	＞6.1 and ＜7.0	＜7.8
Impaired Glucose Tolerance（IGT）	＜6.1	＞7.8 and ＜11.1
IFG+IGT	＞6.1 and ＜7.0	＞7.8 and ＜11.1

A.2 Range of Blood Lipid Marginal Elevation

Referred to *Guidelines of Prevention and Treatment for Dyslipidemia in Adults* (Revised in 2016)by Chinese Association for the Revision of Guidelines for Prevention and Treatment of Dyslipidemia in Adults.

Table A.2　Appropriate and Abnormal Levels of Blood Lipids Stratification Criteria［mmol/L (mg/dl)］

Stratification	TC	LDL-C	HDL-C	non-HDL-C	TG
Ideal Level		＜2.6(100)		＜3.4(130)	
Appropriate Level	＜5.2(200)	＜3.4(130)		＜4.1(160)	＜1.7(150)
Marginal Elevation	≥5.2 (200) and ＜6.2(240)	≥3.4 (130) and ＜4.1(160)		≥4.1 (160) and ＜4.9(190)	≥1.7 (150) and ＜2.3(200)
Elevation	≥6.2(240)	≥4.1(160)		≥4.9(190)	≥2.3(200)
Reduction			＜1.0(40)		

Note：TC, total cholesterol; LDL-C, low density lipoprotein cholesterol; HDL-C, high density lipoprotein cholesterol; non-HDL-C, non-high density lipoprotein cholesterol; TG, triglyceride.

A.3　Diagnostic criteria for non-alcoholic fatty liver

a) No drinking history or alcohol consumption is less than 140 g/week (female < 70 g/week).

b)Excluding viral hepatitis, drug-induced liver disease, total parenteral nutrition, hepatolenticular degeneration, autoimmune liver disease and other specific diseases that can cause fatty liver.

c)Liver biopsy histological changes meet the pathological diagnostic criteria of fatty liver disease, and the activity score < 3 points.

Table A.3 Criteria of liver biopsy to assess NAFLD activity score(NAS)

Pathological changes	Points			
	0 points	1 points	2 points	3 points
Hepatocyte steatosis	< 5%	5%~33%	34%~66%	> 66%
Chronic inflammation in the lobules(20 times microscopic count necrosis)	none	< 2	2~4	> 4
Hepatocyte balloon-like changes	none	rare	common	

Given that the difficult diagnosis of liver histology, non-alcoholic simple fatty liver work is defined as: liver imaging findings meet the diagnostic criteria for diffuse fatty liver and no other reason to explain (Fibro-Touch: 240db/m ⩽ fat attenuation value < 265db/m mild, 265db/m ⩽ fat attenuation value < 295db/m moderate, 295db/m ⩽ fat attenuation value, severe fatty liver), and liver biochemical indicators of normal peripheral blood were normal.

In addition, most patients have a HOMA index of more than 0.5 and IR is present. There may be intestinal flora imbalance, with methane hydrogen exhalation check showing H^2, CH^4 exhalation high peak emerges early or peak increase.

APPENDIX B
(Normative Appendix)
Diagnostic Criteria for Stage Ⅱ of GLMD

B.1 Diagnostic Criteria for Type 2 Diabetes

Referred to *Diagnostic Criteria for Type 2 Diabetes, 1999, WHO.*

Table B.1 WHO Diagnostic Criteria for Type 2 Diabetes, 1999

Diagnostic Criteria	Venous plasma glucose level (mmol/L)
Typical diabetes symptoms (polydipsia,polyphagia, polyuria and weight loss)plus random blood glucose test	$\geqslant 11.1$
or plus	
FPG test	$\geqslant 7.0$
or plus	
Glucose loading test after 2 hours	$\geqslant 11.1$
Those with no symptoms of diabetes should be examined again another day	

Notes:

a. Fasting state refers to no calorie intake for at least 8 hours.

b. Random blood glucose refers to blood sugar at any time of the day cannot be used to diagnose impaired fasting blood glucose or impaired glucose tolerance without consideration of the time of last meal.

c. Glucose loading test after 2 hours: Plasma glucose levels for 2 hours (2h PG) in oral glucose (75g anhydroglucose) tolerance test (OGTT).

d. ADA guidelines in 2010 took HbA1c $\geqslant 6.5\%$ as one of the criteria of diagnostic for diabetes, and WHO recommended that it should be used for diabetes diagnosis in countries and regions with appropriate conditions in 2011. However, HbA1c detection is not common in China and its method has a low degree of standardization, and the study of HbA1c with large Chinese sample is deficient, HbA1c is not recommended for diagnosis of Type 2 DM, but it can be used as a monitoring index for disease treatment.

B.2 Diagnostic Criteria for dyslipidemia

Referred to *Guidelines for the Prevention and treatment of dyslipidemia in Adult in China* (2016 revised edition by Chinese Joint Committee for the Revision of Guidelines for the Prevention and treatment of Lipid Disorders in Adults.

Table B.2   Clinical classification of dyslipidemia

	TC	TG	HDL-C	Equal to types of WHO
Hypercholesterolemia	increase			Ⅱ a
High TG		increase		Ⅳ、Ⅰ
Combined hyperlipemia	increase	increase		Ⅱ b、Ⅲ、Ⅳ、Ⅴ
Low HDL-C			decrease	

Notes: TC, total cholesterol; TG, glycerin trilaurate; HDL-C, high-density lipoprotein cholesterol.

B.2.1   Those who meets any of the following conditions may be directly classified as the ASCVD high-risk group.

a)LDL-C ≥ 4.9mmol/L or TC ≥ 7.2mmol/L.

b)Diabetics with age ≥ 40 years, 1.8mmol/L ≤ LDL-C < 4.9mmol/L, or 3.1mmol/L ≤ TC < 7.2mmol/L.

B.2.2   For individuals who do not have these conditions, the overall risk of ASCVD over the next 10 years should be assessed according to table B.3 below with the consideration if it is needed to get lipid regulation therapy. The average risk of ASCVD in 10 years in different combinations is defined as low risk, moderate risk and high risk according to < 5%, 5%~9%, ≥ 10% respectively.

Table B.3   Risk assessment of ASCVD

	Risk factors*number	level stratification of Serum cholesterol (mmol/L)		
		3.1 ≤ TC < 4.1 or 1.8 ≤ LDL-C < 2.6	4.1 ≤ TC < 5.2 or 2.6 ≤ LDL-C < 3.4	5.2 ≤ TC < 7.2 or 3.4 ≤ LDL-C < 4.9
Without hypertension	0~1	Low risk	Low risk	Low risk
	2	Low risk	Low risk	Moderate risk
	3	Low risk	Moderate risk	Moderate risk
With hypertension	0	Low risk	Low risk	Low risk
	1	Low risk	Moderate risk	Moderate risk
	2	Moderate risk	High risk	High risk
	3	High risk	High risk	High risk

Note: Risk factors include smoking, low HDL-C, male ≥ 45 years or female ≥ 55 years.

B.2.3   Assess the ASCVD risk for the rest of people's life for patient with a moderate ASCVD risk in recent 10 years, and identify individual with high ASCVD risk for the rest life among young and middle-aged people and take action to get early intervention for risk factors which include blood lipids. For the population with moderate ASCVD risk for 10 years, they will have high ASCVD risk for the rest of the life if they meet any of the following 2 or more risk factors. These risk factors include.

a) Systolic pressure ≥ 160mmHg (1mmHg=0.133kPa) or diastolic pressure ≥ 100mmHg.

b) Non-HDL-C $\geqslant$ 5.2mmol/L (200mg/dl).

c) HDL-C $\leqslant$ 1.0mmol/L (40mg/dl).

d) Body Mass Index (BMI) $\geqslant$ 28kg/m2.

e) Smoking.

B.3 Diagnostic criteria of non-alcoholic fatty hepatitis

Based on the diagnosis of non-alcoholic simple fatty liver disease, liver biochemical index is abnormal or liver biopsy evaluation NAS > 4 points accompanied by pre-diabetes or edge hyperlipidemia. HOMA index of most patients is more than 0.5 with the presence of IR. Most of them had intestinal dysbacteriosis, and the peak breath values of H^2 and CH^4 appear earlier or increase according to methane and hydrogen breath test.

APPENDIX C
(Normative Appendix)
Diagnostic Criteria for Stage Ⅲ of GLMD

C.1　Diagnostic Criteria for chronic complications of diabetes mellitus

C.1.1　National Workshop on Microvascular Complications

Referred to *Guidelines for the prevention and treatment of type 2 diabetes in China* (2013 edition)by Chinese Society of Diabetes, Chinese Medical Association.

a) Stage I: glomerular hyperfiltration and increased renal volume.

b) Stage Ⅱ : Intermittent micro albuminuria and normal albumin/creatinine ratio (ACR) at morning or random urine collection when patents have a rest (male<2.5mg/ mmol and female< 3.5mg/mmol) are present. Pathological examination shows slight thickening of glomerular basement membrane (GBM) and slight broadening of mesangial matrix.

c) Stage Ⅲ : Early stage of diabetic nephropathy is marked by persistent microalbuminuria, ACR is 2.5-30.0mg/mmol (male), 3.5-30.0mg/mmol (female). Pathological examination shows that GBM is thickened and mesangial matrix is widened obviously, and hyalinization is present in the Arteriole wall.

d) Stage Ⅳ : Clinical diabetic nephropathy, dominant proteinuria, ACR > 30.0mg/mmol. Some of them are manifested as nephrotic syndrome. Glomerulonephropathy is more serious and partial glomerulosclerosis, focal tubular atrophy and interstitial fibrosis are present according to pathological examination.

e) Stage V: Renal failure stage

Diabetic nephropathy is an important type of chronic renal disease. Non-diabetic nephropathy should be excluded during diagnosis and non-diabetic nephropathy should be considered if the following situations are met: relatively short course of diabetes, simple renal-derived hematuria or proteinuria with hematuria, rapid deterioration of renal function in the short term, without retinopathy, sudden edema and massive proteinuria with normal renal function, significant renal tubular dysfunction, abnormal tubules form with obvious mergence. If it is difficult for differentiation, it can be distinguished by renal biopsy.

C.1.2　Diabetes Retinopathy

Referred to *Diabetic Retinopathy PPP*(2017 edition) by American Academy of Ophthalmology.

Diabetic retinopathy is a highly specific microvascular complication of diabetes and it is the most common cause of new cases with blindness in adults aged 20 to 74 years.Diabetic retinopathy is classified according to indicator that can observe through ophthalmoscope after mydriasis. The international clinical classification of diabetic retinopathy is shown in Table C.1.

Table C.1 International Clinical Classification of Diabetic Retinopathy

Pathological severity level	Manifestations under fundus cope after mydriasis.
No significant diabetic retinopathy	No abnormalities
Mild NPDR	Only microaneurysm
Moderate NPDR	More severe than micro hemangioma, but better than severe NPDR
Severe NPDR	
AAO Definition	Proliferative retinopathy is absent in any of the followings : In each of the four quadrants, severe intra-retinal hemorrhage and micro hemangioma are all present There are obvious string-of-beads changes of veins in two or more quadrants Moderate IRMA is present in one or more quadrants
International Definition	Proliferative retinopathy is absent in any of the following: In each of the four quadrants, there are more than 20 places with intra-retinal hemorrhage in each quadrant. There are obvious string-of-beads changes of veins in two or more quadrants Significant IRMA is present in one or more quadrants
PDR	one or two of the followings are met: neovascularization Vitreous/ retinal hemorrhage

Notes: NPDR, nonproliferative diabetic retinopathy; PDR, proliferative diabetic retinopathy; AAO, American Academy of Ophthalmology.

C.1.3 Diabetes Complicated with Cardiovascular Disease

Risk assessment for coronary heart disease, ask all patients with abnormal glucose metabolism if they have the symptoms of coronary heart disease, and immediate examination and treatment for people with symptoms should be taken.The screening methods for asymptomatic myocardial ischemia include electrocardiography exercise test, dynamic myocardial imaging or stress echocardiography, etc. These tests suggest that patients with asymptomatic myocardial ischemia may perform coronary CT angiography (CTA) and calculate calcification scores, which is helpful to predict prognosis and choose treatment methods.

C.1.4 Diabetes Complicated with Cerebrovascular Disease

In the risk assessment for stroke, diabetes is an independent risk factor for stroke especially ischemic cerebrovascular disease.As with assessment screening principles of coronary heart disease, the risk assessment for stroke emphases on neurological symptoms and signs and appropriate adjuvant examinations which include homocysteine, carotid and transcranial Doppler ultrasound, cranial CT, magnetic resonance imaging and angiography. Some patients need cardiovascular-related tests to screen patients with high-risk of cardiogenic embolism.Diabetics is a high-risk group for carotid artery diseaseswhich is an independent risk factor for stroke, so auscultation of carotid arteries should be regarded as a primary screening method for carotid artery stenosis.With the help of intracranial and extravascular ultrasound, CT or magnetic resonance imaging and angiography, asymptomatic carotid artery diseases or asymptomatic cerebral infarction in patients with diabetes should be detected early.

C.1.5 Diabetes Complicated with Peripheral Vascular Diseases

Referred to *Guidelines for the prevention and treatment of type 2 diabetes in China* (2017 edition), by Chinese Society of Diabetes, Chinese Medical Association.

Diabetic peripheral vascular diseases usually refer to peripheral artery disease (PAD) which is caused by the atherosclerosis of lower extremity blood vessels, leading to the artery stenosis, the occlusion, and even necrosis of distal lower extremity tissue in serious cases.As a sign of systemic arteriosclerosis, PAD often coexists with other major vascular complications. The diagnosis should meet the following criteria.

a) If resting ankle brachial index (ABI) of patent is equal or less than 0.90, no matter the symptom of lower extremity discomfort exists or not.

b)Patients with lower extremity discomfort and resting ABI $\geqslant$ 0.90 during exercise, such as ABI decreases by 15% -20% after treadmill test;Severe limb ischemia should be diagnosed if resting ABI < 0. 40 or ankle arterial pressure < 50mmHg or toe arterial pressure < 30 mm Hg.

C.1.6 Distal Symmetric Polyneuropathy of Diabetes

Referred to *Guidelines for the prevention and treatment of type 2 diabetes in China* (2017 edition) by Chinese Society of Diabetes, Chinese Medical Association.

C.1.6.1 Criteria of diagnosis for distal symmetric polyneuropathy of diabetes mellitus

a) A clear history of diabetes is present.

b) Neuropathy is present during or after diagnosis of diabetes.

c)The clinical symptoms and signs are consistent with the manifestation of distal symmetric diabetic polyneuropathy of diabetes.

d) For patients with clinical symptoms (pain, numbness, abnormal sensation, etc.), any of the 5 examinations (ankle reflex, sensation for acupuncture pain, vibration, pressure and temperature) is abnormal.

e) For patients without clinical symptoms, if 2 of the 5 tests were abnormal, they will be diagnosed as distal symmetric polyneuropathy clinically.

C.1.6.2 Excluded diagnosis of distal symmetric polyneuropathy in diabetes

a) Other causes for neuropathy, such as cervical and lumbar spondylosis (nerve root compression, spinal canal stenosis, cervical and lumbar degeneration), cerebral infarction, and Guillain-Barre syndrome should be excluded.

b) Severe arteriovenous vascular diseases, such as venous embolism, lymphangitis should be excluded.

c) It is still necessary to distinguish neurotoxicity caused by drugs, especially chemotherapeutic drugs, and the nerve damage caused by renal insufficiency leading to metabolic toxicants.

d)Patients who need diagnosis can be examined by electromyography.

C.1.6.3 Clinical diagnostic classification of distal symmetric polyneuropathy in diabetes

C.1.6.3.1 Diagnosis: symptoms or signs of distal symmetric polyneuropathy and abnormal nerve function in conduction are present.

C.1.6.3.2 Clinical diagnosis: the symptoms of distal symmetric polyneuropathy are present and one sign is positive, or the symptom is absent but more than 2 (include 2) signs is positive.

C.1.6.3.3 Suspected: symptoms of distal symmetric polyneuropathy are present but without signs, or symptom is absent but one sign is positive;

C.1.6.3.4 Subclinical: no symptoms and signs, only abnormal nerve function in conduction.

C.1.6.4 Diabetic Autonomic Neuropathy

C.1.6.4.1 Cardiovascular autonomic neuropathy: the manifestations include orthostatic hypotension, syncope, abnormal coronary systolic and diastolic function, painless myocardial infarction, cardiac arrest or sudden death.There is no unified diagnostic standard at present. The examinations include heart rate variability, Valsalva test, fist grip test (blood pressure measurement after gripping for 3 minutes), postural blood pressure measurement, 24-hour ambulatory blood pressure monitoring, and spectrum analysis and so on.

C.1.6.4.2 Autonomic neuropathy of digestive system: the manifestations include dysphagia, hiccup, upper abdomen fullness, stomach discomfort, constipation, diarrhea and defecation. The examinations which include electrogastrogram, esophageal manometry, scintillation scan for gastric emptying (measurement of the time of solid and liquid food emptying) and electrophysiological examination for local peripheral neuropathy of rectum can be used for diagnosis.

C.1.6.4.3 Autonomic neuropathy in urogenital system: The clinical manifestations include urinary disorders: urinary retention, urinary incontinence, urinary tract infection, hyposexuality, erectile dysfunction, menstrual disorder and so on.Ultrasound can test bladder volume, residual urine volume and nerve conduction velocity can test urethral-nerve function in diabetes.

C.1.6.4.4 Other autonomic neuropathy: for example, abnormal temperature regulation and sweating is manifested as less or no sweating, which leads to dry hands and feet cracking and secondary infection.In addition, because low capillary tension cause vein dilatation, it is easy to form "micro hemangioma" locally and get secondary infection. Lack of normal perception of hypoglycemia, etc.

C.1.7 Diagnosis of Diabetic Lower Extremity Vascular Diseases

Referred to *Guidelines for the prevention and treatment of type 2 diabetes in China* (2017 edition) by Chinese Society of Diabetes, Chinese Medical Association.

a)Meet the criteria of diagnosis for diabetes.

b)Clinical manifestation of lower extremity ischemia is present.

c)The auxiliary examinations show the presence of the lower extremity vascular disease. Rest ABI<0.9 or rest ABI>0.9, but lower extremity discomfort occurred during exercise and ABI decreased by 15%~20% after treadmill test or imaging indicates the presence of vascular stenosis.

C.1.8 Diagnosis of diabetic peripheral neuropathy

Referred to *Guidelines for the prevention and treatment of type 2 diabetes in China* (2017 edition) by Chinese Society of Diabetes, Chinese Medical Association.

a) A clear history of diabetes is present.

b) Neuropathy occurs during or after the diagnosis of diabetes.

c) Clinical symptoms and signs are consistent with the manifestations of diabetic peripheral neuropathy.

d) If people are abnormal at two or more of the following 5 examinations, they are diagnosed as diabetic peripheral neuropathy.

1) Abnormal perception for temperature.

2) Monofilament examination, sensation on food loses or disappears.

3) Abnormal sense for vibration.

4) Ankle reflex disappears.

5) Nerve conduction velocity slowed down in 2 or more items.

C.2 Acute Coronary Syndrome（ACS）

Acute coronary syndrome (ACS) is a group of clinical syndrome based on rupture or invasion of coronary atherosclerotic plaque and secondary complete or incomplete occlusive thrombosis in pathologically, which include acute ST elevation myocardial infarction (STEMI), acute non-ST elevation myocardial infarction (NSTEMI) and unstable angina (UA). The diagnostic criteria are as follows.

Table C.2 Classification and diagnostic criteria for ACS

Classification for ACS	Diagnostic Criteria
STEMI	The electrocardiogram shows that ST segment is arched and raised upward, which is accompanied by one or more following situation: persistent ischemic chest pain (with the duration more than 30 minutes and cannot be alleviated by Sublingual administration of nitroglycerin); echocardiogram shows regional wall motion abnormality; coronary arteriography is abnormal.
NSTEMI	$cTn>99^{th}ULN$ or $CK\text{-}MB>99^{th}ULN$, accompanied by one or more following situations: persistent ischemic chest pain (with the duration more than 30 minutes and cannot be alleviated by sublingual administration of nitroglycerin); The electrocardiogram shows that new ST segment is depressed or T wave was low and inverted; echocardiogram shows regional wall motion abnormality; coronary arteriography is abnormal;
UA	Negative cTn, ischemic chest pain(new onset or more frequent than before, prolonged duration, aggravated severity, or onset at rest and at night),electrocardiogram showed transient ST segment is depression or T wave is low or inverted, elevated ST segment is rare(variant angina)

Notes：cTn, cardiac troponin; CK-MB, creatinine kinase- MB; ULN, Upper limit of normal reference value; the electrocardiogram shows that ST segment is arched and raised upward; ST segment is arched and raised upward after J points in two adjacent lead(V2-V3 lead $\geqslant$ 0.25mV(<40 years for male) $\geqslant$ 0.20mV($\geqslant$ 40 years for male) or $\geqslant$ 0.15mV(female), other adjacent chest leads or limb leads $\geqslant$ 0.1mV with or without decreased pathological Q wave and R wave.

C.3 Stable angina

a) With the history of typical angina of effort for more than half a year.

b) Changes of ST-T in electrocardiogram during onset.

c) Coronary angiogram shows that at least one vessel has more than 50% of fixed stenosis.

C.4 Acute ischemic stroke (acute cerebral infarction)

a) Acute onset.

b) The focal nerve function is impaired (unilateral facial or physical weakness or numbness, speech disorders, etc.), and comprehensive nerve function is impaired in a few cases.

c)The time duration of symptoms or signs is unlimited (when the imaging shows that the ischemic focus that is responsible for the disease is present) or more than 24 hours (when the imaging shows that the ischemic focus that is responsible for the disease is absent based on imaging).

d)Non-vascular etiology is excluded.

e) Intracerebral Hemorrhage is excluded based on brain CT or MRI.

C.5 Transient ischemic attack (TIA)

Transient neurological dysfunction caused by focal ischemia of the brain, spinal cord, or retina without acute cerebral infarction.

C.6 Peripheral artery disease (PAD)

PAD refers to arterial diseases other than coronary and intracranial arteries diseases, which include stenosis, occlusion and aneurysm. These diseases are mainly associated with arteriosclerosis, chronic inflammation, hereditary dysplasia, and traumatic peripheral artery disease account for only 5%~10% of all PAD cases.

C.7 Diagnostic criteria of non-alcoholic fatty cirrhosis

a) With a history of non-alcoholic simple fatty liver disease.

b) Type-B ultrasound and / or CT examination showed liver cirrhosis or Fibro-Touch examination showed 11.9 kPA of liver hardness, or microscope for liver biopsy shows pseudo lobules formation and fibrous tissue proliferation.

c)Patients at this stage may have overgrowth of enteric bacterial accompanied with impaired barrier function of intestine.

C.8 Diagnostic Criteria of Arteriosclerosis Obliterans in Lower Extremities

ASO clinical diagnosis for lower extremity can be made if first 4 diagnostic criteria are met.

a) Age > 40 years.

b) Smoking, diabetes, hypertension, hyperlipidemia and other high risk factors are present.

c) Clinical manifestation of arteriosclerosis obliterans in lower extremities is present.

d) Ischemic distal arterial pulse decreases or disappears.

e) ABI $\leq$ 0.9.

f) Color Doppler ultrasound, CTA, MRA and DSA showed the stenosis or occlusion of the artery.

Bibliography

[1] The State Bureau of Technical Supervision. Technical terms for clinical diagnosis and treatment of traditional Chinese medicine—Diseases〔S〕. Beijing : Standards Press of China, GB/T16751.1—1997.

[2] The State Bureau of Technical Supervision. Technical terms for clinical diagnosis and treatment of traditional Chinese medicine—Syndromes〔S〕. Beijing : Standards Press of China, GB/T16751.2—1997.

[3] The State Bureau of Technical Supervision. Technical terms for clinical diagnosis and treatment of traditional Chinese medicine—Therapeutic methods〔S〕. Beijing : Standards Press of China, GB/T16751.3—1997.

[4] China Association of Chinese Medicine. Guidelines for diagnosis and treatment of common internal diseases in traditional Chinese medicine—TCM diseases and symptoms〔S〕. Beijing :China Press of Traditional Chinese Medicine, ZYYXH/T41—2008.

[5] China Association of Chinese Medicine. Guidelines for diagnosis and treatment of common internal diseases in traditional Chinese medicine—Western diseases〔S〕. Beijing :China Press of Traditional Chinese Medicine ,ZYYXH/T50-135—2008.

[6] China Association of Chinese Medicine. Guidelines for diabetes prevention and control of traditional Chinese medicine Part of diabetes and its complications〔S〕. Beijing: China Press of Traditional Chinese Medicine, ZYYXH/T3.1-15—2007.

[7] Guo Jiao, Xiao Xue, Rong Xianglu, et al. Glucolipid Metabolic Disease and precision medicine〔J〕. World Science and Technology/Modernization of Traditional Chinese Medicine and Materia Medica, 2017, 19(1):50-54.

[8] Guo Jiao. Research progress on prevention and treatment of Glucolipid Metabolic Disease with integrated traditional Chinese and Western medicine〔J〕. Chinese Journal of Integrative Medicine, 2017, 23(6):403-409.

[9] International Diabetes Federation. IDF Diabetes Atlas.8th ed.〔EB/OL〕. https://www.idf.org/e-library/welcome.html,2017/2018-09-10.

[10] Wang L,Gao P, Zhang M,et al.Prevalence and Ethnic Pattern of Diabetes and Prediabetes in China in 2013〔J〕. JAMA,2017,317(24):2515-2523.

[11] Department of disease prevention and control of national health and family planning commission. Report on Nutrition and chronic Diseases of Chinese residents (2015)〔R〕. Beijing: People's Medical Publishing House, 2015.

[12] Moran A,Gu D,Zhao D,et al. Future Cardiovascular Disease in China: Markov Model and Risk Factor Scenario Projections From the Coronary Heart Disease Policy Model-China〔J〕.Circulation:Cardiovascular Quality and Outcomes,2010, 3(3):243-252.

[13] Younossi ZM,Koenig AB,Abdelatif D,et al. Global epidemiology of nonalcoholic fatty liver disease-Meta-analytic assessment of prevalence, incidence, and outcomes〔J〕. Hepatology, 2016, 64(1):73-84.

[14] Xiang Lei, Piao Shenghua, Rong Xianglu,et al. Analysis of the distribution of syndrome of Damp-Heat Syndrome〔J〕.World Chinese Medicine, 2018,13(10):2621-2624.

[15] Chinese Society of Diabetes, Chinese Medical Association. Guidelines for the prevention and treatment of type 2 diabetes in China〔M〕. Beijing: Peking University Medical Press, 2014.

［16］ Fang Chaohui, Tong Xiaoling, DuanJungu, et al. Clinical practice guidelines for evidence-based traditional Chinese Medicine in prediabetes ［J］. Journal of Traditional Chinese Medicine, 2017, 58(3):266-270.

［17］ Chinese Society of Diabetes, China Association of Chinese Medicine. Standard of TCM diagnosis and treatment of diabetes complicated with metabolic syndrome ［J］. World Journal of Integrated Traditional and Western Medicine, 2011, 06(2):177-179.

［18］ Chinese Joint Committee for the Revision of Guidelines for the Prevention and treatment of Lipid Disorders in Adults. Guidelines for the Prevention and treatment of dyslipidemia in Adult in China (2016 revised edition)［J］. Chinese Circulation Journal, 2016, 16(10):15-35.

［19］ Professional Group of Atherosclerosis and Dyslipidemia, Cardiovascular Disease Committee of Chinese Association of the integration of Traditional and Western Medicine. Expert consensus on the diagnosis and treatment of dyslipidemia by combination of traditional Chinese and western medicine ［J］. Chinese General Practice, 2017, 20(3):262-269.

［20］ National Workshop on Fatty Liver and Alcoholic Liver Disease, Chinese Society of Hepatology, Chinese Medical Association. Guidelines for prevention and treatment of nonalcoholic fatty liver disease (2018 update)［J］. Journal of Clinical Hepatology, 2018, 21(2):177-186.

［21］ Spleen and Stomach Disease Branch, China Association of Chinese Medicine. Expert consensus on TCM diagnosis and treatment of nonalcoholic fatty liver disease (2017)［J］. Journal of Traditional Chinese Medicine, 2017, 58(19):1706-1710.

［22］ Chalasani N,Younossi Z,Lavine JE,et al.The diagnosis and management of non-alcoholic fatty liver disease: practice Guideline by the American Association for the Study of Liver Diseases,American College of Gastroenterology,and the American Gastroenterological Association ［J］.Hepatology,2012,55(6):2005-2023.

［23］ Wong VW,Chan WK,Chitturi S,et al.Asia-Pacific Working Party on Non-alcoholic Fatty Liver Disease guidelines 2017-Part 1: Definition,risk factors and assessment ［J］.J Gastroenterol Hepatol,2018,33(1):70-85.

［24］ Robinson JG,Stone NJ.The 2013 ACC/AHA guideline on the treatment of blood cholesterol to reduce atherosclerotic cardiovascular disease risk: a new paradigm supported by more evidence ［J］.Eur Heart J,2015,36(31):2110-2118.

［25］ Shi Dazhuo. Diagnostic criteria of coronary heart disease with blood stasis syndrome［J］. Chinese journal of integrated traditional and western medicine, 2016, 36(10):1162-1162.

［26］ Emergency Physicians Branch, Chinese Physicians Association. Guidelines for rapid diagnosis and treatment with emergency of acute coronary syndrome ［J］. Chinese journal of critical care medicine, 2016, 25(4):397-404.

［27］ Group of drafting guidelines for the diagnosis and treatment of acute ischemic stroke, national workshop on cerebrovascular disease, Chinese society of hepatology, Chinese medical association. Guidelines for the diagnosis and treatment of acute ischemic stroke in China 2010 ［J］. Chinese Journal of Neurology, 2010, 43(2):146-153.

［28］ Beijing center for quality control and improvement of diagnosis and treatment of stroke. Criteria for screening and diagnosis of Cerebral Atherosclerosis (2014 edition)-applicable for general hospital in Beijing (secondary and tertiary medical institutions) applicable［J］. National Medical Journal of China, 2014,94(47):3705-3711.

［29］ An Dongqing, Wu Zonggui. Expert consensus on the diagnosis and treatment of atherosclerosis by combination of traditional chinese and western medicine [J] . Chinese General Practice, 2017, 20(5):507-511.

[30] National workshop on vascular surgery, Chinese society of surgery, Chinese medical association. Guidelines for the diagnosis and treatment of carotid artery stenosis [J] . Chinese Journal of Vascular Surgery (Electronic Version), 2017,9(3) :169-175.

[31] National drafting workshop on expert's suggestions for diagnosis and treatment of atherosclerotic renal artery stenosis. Chinese expert recommendations for management of atherosclerotic renal artery stenosis (2010) [J] . Chinese Journal of Geriatrics, 2010, 29(4):265-270.

[32] National workshop on vascular surgery, Chinese society of surgery, Chinese medical association. Guidelines for the diagnosis and treatment of lower extremity arteriosclerosis obliterans (volume one) [J] . National Medical Journal of China, 2015, 7(3):145-151.

[33] Zheng Xiaoyu. Guidance principle of clinical study on new drug of traditional Chinese medicine(proposed) [M] . Beijing: The Medicine Science and Technology Press of China,2002.

[34] Zhai H L, Wang N J, Han B, et al. Low vitamin D levels and non-alcoholic fatty liver disease, evidence for their independent association in men in East China: a cross-sectional study (Survey on Prevalence in East China for Metabolic Diseases and Risk Factors (SPECT-China)) [J] . British Journal of Nutrition, 2016, 115(8): 1352-1359.

[35] Bovet P,Chiolero A,Gedeon J.Health Effects of Overweight and Obesity in 195 Countries [J] .N Engl J Med,2017,377(15):1495-1496.

[36] World Health Organization,A global brief on Hypertension [EB/OL] . https://www.who.int/ cardiovascular_ diseases/publications/global_brief_ hypertension/zh,2013/2018-10-14.

[37] Wang Z,Chen Z,Zhang L,et al.Status of Hypertension in China: Results from the China Hypertension Survey,2012-2015 [J] .Circulation, 2018,137(22):2344-2356.

[38] Yu X,Tian X,Wang S.Age-specific relevance of usual blood pressure to vascular mortality: a meta-analysis of individual data for one million adults in 61 propective studies [J] .Journal of the Lepidopterists Society,2002,52(26):141-147.

[39] Pu Shenghua, GuoJiao, HuXingping. Clinical Research of Chinese Medicine Syndromes of Hyperlipidemia Inpatients [J] . Chinese Journal of Traditional Chinese Medicine and Pharmacy, 2012, 32(10):1322-1325.

[40] Ji L,Hu D,Pan C,et al.Primacy of the 3B approach to control risk factors for cardiovascular disease in type 2 diabetes patients [J] . Am J Med,2013,126(10): 925.e11-22.

[41] Liver and Alcoholic Liver Disease, Chinese Society of Hepatology, Chinese Medical Association. Guidelines of prevention and treatment for nonalcoholic fatty liver disease(2018 update) [J] . Journal of Practical Hepatopathy, 2018,21(2) 177-186.

[42] Portillo-Sanchez P,Bril F,Maximos M,et al.High Prevalence of Nonalcoholic Fatty Liver Disease in Patients With Type 2 Diabetes Mellitus and Normal Plasma Aminotransferase Levels [J] .J Clin Endocrinol Metab,2015,100(6):2231-2238.

[43] Leite NC,Villela-Nogueira CA,Pannain VL,et al.Histopathological stages of nonalcoholic fatty liver disease in type 2 diabetes: prevalences and correlated factors [J] .Liver Int,2011,31(5):700-706.

[44] Targher G,Bertolini L,Rodella S,et al.Non-alcoholic fatty liver disease is independently associated with an increased prevalence of chronic kidney disease and proliferative/laser-treated retinopathy in type 2 diabetic patients [J] .Diabetologia,2008,51(3):444-450.

[45] Zhao Y,Sun H,Wang B,et al.Impaired fasting glucose predicts the development of hypertension over

6 years in female adults: Results from the rural Chinese cohort study ［J］.J Diabetes Complicatio ns,2017,31(7):1090-1095.

［46］ Emdin CA,Anderson SG,Woodward M,et al. Usual Blood Pressure and Risk of New-Onset Diabetes: Evidence From 4.1 Million Adults and a Meta-Analysis of Prospective Studies ［J］.J Am Coll Cardiol,2015,66(14):1552-1562.

［47］ Zhang Y,Jiang X,Bo J,et al.Risk of stroke and coronary heart disease among various levels of blood pressure in diabetic and nondiabetic Chinese patients ［J］.J Hypertens,2018,36(1):93-100.

［48］ Pan L,Yang Z,Wu Y,et al.The prevalence,awareness,treatment and control of dyslipidemia among adults in China ［J］.Atherosclerosis,2016,248:2-9.

［49］ Pan H,Guo J,Su Z.Advances in understanding the interrelations between leptin resistance and obesity ［J］. Physiol Behav,2014,130:157-169.

［50］ Zhang Jingjing. Study on the effect and mechanism of compound Zhenzhu Tiaozhi recipe on improving glucose and lipid metabolism based on HPA Axis［D］. Guangzhou:Guangdong Pharmaceutical University, 2017.

［51］ Ye DW,Rong XL,Xu AM,et al.Liver-adipose tissue crosstalk: A key player in the pathogenesis of glucolipid metabolic disease ［J］.Chin J Integr Med,2017,23(6):410-414.

［52］ Ding C,Guo J,Su Z.The status of research into resistance to diet-induced obesity ［J］.Horm Metab Res,2015,47(6):404-410.

［53］ Saltiel AR,Kahn CR.Insulin signalling and the regulation of glucose and lipid metabolism ［J］. Nature,2001,414(6865):799-806.

［54］ Liu J,Zhuang ZJ,Bian DX,et al.Toll-like receptor-4 signalling in the progression of non-alcoholic fatty liver disease induced by high-fat and high-fructose diet in mice ［J］.Clin Exp Pharmacol Physiol,2014,41(7):482-488.

［55］ Corkey BE.Banting lecture 2011: hyperinsulinemia: cause or consequence［J］. Diabetes, 2012,61(1):4-13.

［56］ Wei Zhifu. Study on the effect and mechanism of FTZ on improving glucose and lipid metabolism induced by persistent inflammation［D］. Guangzhou:Guangdong Pharmaceutical University, 2017.

［57］ Li M,Han Z,Bei W,et al.Oleanolic Acid Attenuates Insulin Resistance via NF-κB to Regulate the IRS1-GLUT4 Pathway in HepG2 Cells ［J］.Evid Based Complement Alternat Med,2015:643102.

［58］ Glass CK,Olefsky JM.Inflammation and lipid signaling in the etiology of insulin resistance ［J］.Cell Metab,2012,15(5):635-645.

［59］ Yuan Yu, Sui Zhimei, Zhangyang, et al. Effects of intestinal micro ecology on the pathogenesis and treatment of non-alcoholic fatty liver disease ［J］. Chinese Journal of Hepatology, 2016, 24(5):375-379.

［60］ Zhong HJ,Yuan Y,Xie WR,et al.Type 2 Diabetes Mellitus Is Associated with More Serious Small Intestinal Mucosal Injuries ［J］.PLoS One,2016,11(9):e0162354.

［61］ Zhong Haojie, Wu Lihao, Chen Yu, et al. Metabolic syndrome is associated with more serious small intestinal mucosal injury ［J］. World Chinese Journal of Digestology, 2016(11):1754-1759.

［62］ Lu Yuan, Luo Tingting, Yan Shikai, et al. Metabolomics Research Progress in Hyperlipidemia［J］. Guangdong Chemical Industry,2018,45(10):133-135.

［63］ Wang Lusha, Kou Tianshun, Huang Yuncui, et al. Prevention and treatment of non-alcoholic fatty liver by regulating the composition of liver fatty acid with compound Zhenzhu tiaozhi recipe ［J］. World Science and Technology/ Modernization of Traditional Chinese Medicine and Materia Medica, 2018, 20(5):734-743.

［64］ Zhao Huimin, Lei Zili, Guo Jiao. Advances of the contradictory relationship between plasma adiponectin level and type 2 diabetes mellitus and cardiovascular disease [J].Chinese Journal of Cell Biology,2018,40(5):820-826.

[65] Liu Qian, Yin Zhiwei, Duan Shuwei, et al. Development and application of TCM syndrome differentiation guidelines for diabetic nephropathy [J]. Chinese Journal of Kidney Disease Investigation (Electronic Edition), 2018, 7(2): 91-93.

[66] Huang Jingwen, Pu Shenghua, Guo Jiao. Analysis on traditional Chinese medicine constitution types and tongue and pulse [J]. China Journal of Traditional Chinese Medicine and Pharmacy, 2018,33(3):1082-1084.

[67] Li Yu, Xiang Lei, Xiao Xue, et al. Information mining of damp-heat syndrome based on clinical research [J]. Journal of Guangdong Pharmaceutical University,2017,33(5):654-658.

[68] Zhang Xia, Wang Yujiao, Zeng Zhihuan, et al. The Effect of Tianhuang Pian on Intimal Hyperplasia after Vascular Endothelial Injury [J]. Traditional Chinese Drug Research and Clinical Pharmacology, 2017,28(5):606-610.

[69] Sun Yue, Lian Tian, Guo Jiao. Research advances in the sphingosine kinase signaling pathway in liver fibrosis [J]. Journal of Clinical Hepatology, 2017,33(9):1798-1801.

[70] Fu Rong, Rong Xianglu, Guo Jiao. Effect of compound Zhenzhu tiaozhi recipe on liver PPAR α and its downstream gene in non-alcoholic fatty live [J]. Chinese Journal of Traditional Chinese Medicine and Pharmacy. 2017,37(6):735-740.

[71] Wei Zhifu, Lei Zili, Guo Jiao. Research Progress of the Inflammation Mechanism in Hyperglycemia [J]. Pharmacy Today, 2017,27(5):358-360.

[72] Su Shuo, Su Shina, Pu Shenghua, et al. Investigation and Analysis of TCM constitution of College students in Guangzhou [J]. Chinese Journal of Traditional Chinese Medicine and Pharmacy, 2017, 32(4):1833-1835.

[73] Zhang Jingjing, Cai Jinyan, Guo Jiao. Progress on 11β-Hydroxy Steroid Dehydrogenase Type 1 in Type 2 Diabetes Mellitus [J]. Food and Dretcug,2017,19(2):142-147.